"An entire sea of water can't sink
a ship unless it gets inside the ship.
Similarly, the negativity of the world
can't put you down unless you
allow it to get inside you."

~ Goi Nasu

to
TIM!
IN APPRECIATION OF
ALL YOUR HARD WORK!
♡

Within

Compiled by Michael Harris
Foreword by Rajashree Choudhury

Includes:

Dr. Adam Chipiuk
Adrianne "Alax" Jackson
Amy Kreminski
Angelica Daniele and Zeb Homison
Anurag Choudhury
Dr. Avi Sharma
Balwan Singh
Brad Colwell
BridrettAne Goddard
Bynay Blosberg
Cat Koo
Danelle Denstone
Deborah Small
Donna Rubin
Donna Wikio
Emily & Eddie Garner
Gretchen Olsen
John Salvatore
Judy Louie
Kay Forrester
Leo Eisenstein
Mica Fish
Michele Vennard
Nadine Faitas
Rowena Jayne
Spencer Larson

Within

Copyright @ 2023 Michael Harris

Print ISBN: 978-1-666402-49-0

Ebook ISBN: 978-1-666402-48-3

Dedication

Emmy Cleaves
1928 - 2022

"Think young, act young, feel young."

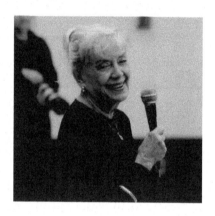

This book is dedicated to the ageless and remarkable Emmy Cleaves.

Emmy, an Eastern European native of Latvia, spent the entirety of World War II as a prisoner in a Nazi slave labor camp. She said, "Fighting is what makes you stronger, more capable, and in some ways, it makes life more thrilling. You become stronger through struggle." Years later, she finally acknowledged that she might not have recovered from a crippling brain aneurysm without Yoga. She claimed that each of such encounters "helped shape me into the person that I am today."

Words cannot express enough our deepest gratitude for all that you have given to the greater Yoga community and to those who have been touched by your endless inspiration to move beyond fear. Everyone in this book and countless more, have had the privilege of being guided by your insights and love of yoga.

You are a true legend, and we're honored to have had the opportunity to learn from you.

CONTENTS

ESSAY FOUR

ESSAY FIVE

ESSAY SIX

ESSAY SEVEN

ESSAY EIGHT

ESSAY NINE

ESSAY TEN

ESSAY EIGHTEEN

ESSAY NINETEEN

ESSAY TWENTY

ESSAY TWENTY-ONE

ESSAY TWENTY-TWO

ESSAY TWENTY-THREE

ESSAY TWENTY-FOUR

ESSAY TWENTY-FIVE

ESSAY TWENTY-SIX

Gratitude & Acknowledgements

The creation of this book, Within, would not have been possible without the support and contributions of many individuals and organizations. I would like to take this opportunity to express my sincere gratitude to each of them.

First and foremost, I want to thank Higher Power, who has guided all the authors and myself on this journey and continues to inspire us to look *within* and live a life of service and love.

I am grateful to Heather Andrews (aka The Compilation Queen) and her team at Get You Published, including Jennifer Traynor for their expert guidance and support in bringing this book to life. Your dedication in helping authors share their messages with the world is truly remarkable.

I also want to extend my heartfelt thanks to Mary Ellen Tribby, CEO at Centerpointe Research Institute, and Larry Michel, Founder of The Institute of Genetic Energetics, for believing in this project and becoming launch partners. In addition, deep gratitude to Balwan Singh of YogaTalk to making his platform a place for all the co-authors to share their message. Your support and encouragement have been invaluable.

I am deeply appreciative of my friend and business partner, Sean Tyler Foley, for always encouraging me to speak my truth and get my message to the world. Your unwavering support means the world to me.

I want to thank David Hancock at Morgan James Publishing for taking a chance on me in 2012 and being my first publisher. Your guidance and expertise over the years, have been instrumental in helping me achieve my dream of becoming a multiple bestselling published author.

To all my yoga teachers, including Erich Shiffman, Nischala Joy Devi, Rajashree Choudhury, Emmy Cleaves, and Bikram Choudhury. I am forever grateful for your wisdom and guidance in discovering my truth. In your own unique way, each of you, have played a significant role in my personal growth and development. It's an honor to have had the privilege of learning from you.

In addition, I would like to express my deep gratitude to Rajashree Choudhury for her unwavering support and belief in me, as well as for graciously providing the foreword for this book.

Last but not least, I want to express my appreciation to each of the phenomenal co-authors for sharing their experiences and insights, and to the readers who have taken the time to read this book. It is my hope that Within will inspire you to look inside and discover the answers you need to live your best life.

Thank you, from the bottom of my heart.

With gratitude,

Michael Harris

**"Where there is love,
there is life."**

- Mahatma Gandhi

FOREWORD

Rajashree Choudhury

Yoga - A Journey of Self-Discovery

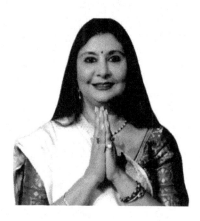

My journey with yoga asanas began at the tender age of four, encouraged by my parents. Growing up in India in the 1970s, it was unusual for boys to participate in yoga classes alongside girls. I eagerly anticipated afternoons spent on the grass, practicing yoga and playing with other children. Running and talking to everyone, I found joy in these shared moments. It was during a demonstration in 1972 that my passion for Yoga truly ignited. I discovered the beauty of moving my body in ways I had never imagined possible. I even won a national challenge trophy, charting a destiny I could have never foreseen.

When I moved to the USA at the age of 20, Yoga continued to play a pivotal role in my life. Throughout my past, present, and future, Yoga has remained an invisible, yet powerful, source of inspiration, offering challenges and solutions from within. By following the eightfold path of Yoga, I have learned to see my successes and failures as transference and countertransference, cultivating a sense of equanimity.

Embracing Equanimity Through Yoga

Today, Yoga is an integral part of my life, bringing balance and inner peace. I highly recommend this compilation book to anyone seeking to delve deeper into the world of Yoga. The 26 contributing authors pour their hearts and souls into sharing how Yoga has touched their lives and made a difference. Each author comes from a unique psychosocial background with diverse faiths and lifestyles. Some may use Yoga as a means to advance their career, while others focus on personal growth. Regardless of their individual paths, Yoga consistently creates positive change for those who commit to practice and trust in the process.

Whether you are a seasoned practitioner or new to Yoga, this book offers the opportunity to connect with 26 extraordinary authors who are all Yoga practitioners and teachers. Each shares their joys, pains, and unique connections to Yoga, and I am confident that you will find resonance with their life stories. As you immerse yourself in these pages, you, too, may discover the transformative power of Yoga that lies Within.

Who's Rajashree?

Rajashree Choudhury began her life in Yoga at the early age of four years. Since then, she dedicated herself to the practice and propagation of Yoga, which, consequently, motivated her towards a multi-facet career as a Yoga instructor, therapist, writer, motivational speaker, philanthropist, and an ardent advocate for children and women.

Born and raised in Kolkata, she moved to Los Angeles at the age of nineteen. Rajashree's background is a true blend of the East and West. Rajashree is a five-time winner of the National Indian Yoga Championship from 1979 to 1983. By age 11, she won several titles. This experience shaped her life's dream of encouraging youth to practice yoga.

To learn more about Rajashree Choudury, visit www.innerpointe.com

"Sometimes when you are in a dark place you think you have been buried, but actually, you have been planted."

~ Christine Caine

Introduction
Michael Harris
Part One
Where It All Started

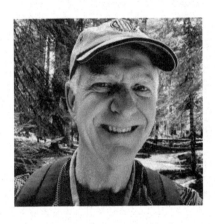

In life, everyone one of us has unexpected events happen. It's as if one day everything is different. Perhaps your life can be like a dumpster fire. A relationship ends, health disintegrates, financial woes set in, a job ends abruptly, or you simply get a flat tire. On the other side, raging success could be the order of the day. New relationships begin, money falls from the sky, a new job (or business) comes along, or we finally are able to get our dream car.

It's all part of this amazing journey of life.

Of course, much of life is out of our control. Day changes to night and the moon replaces the sun. What about that guy that cuts you off in traffic and doesn't even realize it? I don't know about you, but it can be tempting to lash out in uncontrollable anger.

What this book is about is YOUR life and how YOU live it, with a bit of fun, humor and grace mixed in.

You'll discover in the pages that follow how 26 everyday people, by going *within*, found something that gave them a new remarkable life. Some of them experienced unspeakable events, near-death health issues, broken families, or financial despair. Virtually, every tragedy happened. Yet, each one of our co-authors, came out the other side stronger, wiser, and more resilient.

Some of the authors simply wanted to feel better. Then, as life swirled around them, they discovered something unexpected. They realized that their true power was *within* and they could turn this power on at any time. *The secret to life was within them the whole time.*

But wait, I'm getting ahead of the story.

As for me, well, I'm just the lead author and lover of the power of nature. I didn't write an essay for this book - mainly because each of the co-author's words are extremely powerful. But I did want to share a bit of my own journey, as well as some thoughts on ways to find your own answers in life.

So, sit back, grab a cup of tea (or whatever suits your fancy), and let's dive in.

The first thirty years of my life were pretty messy. Don't get me wrong, my parents were wonderful people and did everything to keep me on the straight and narrow. Up until 12 years old, I was on top of the world. My father was an entrepreneur, and my mom was a dedicated housewife. I loved baseball, golf, and chasing trout and crawdads in the nearby creek. Life was good.

Then, in 1971 at 12 years old, tragedy struck. While waterskiing with my brother and friends, I attempted a beach landing with a huge smack. At first, the local hospital said I was just bruised and beat up, and that I would be fine. But 48 hours later, the surgeons took out 60% of my liver and my gallbladder. In addition, I had a half dozen cracked ribs, a collapsed lung and went through 21 blood transfusions. As I slid into a 10-day coma, I wasn't expected to live. After a near-death experience and a talk with the spirits, I woke up suddenly asking for my bike.

Becoming a teenager was confusing. My recovery from the accident was ongoing for about a year. I was that sick-looking kid in school, and I didn't think anyone would like me. It was difficult to be the same playful kid I was used to and at the same time, I was beginning to like the girls. Yet, my self-esteem was in the dumps. By high school, alcohol and drugs became my higher power. Drinking helped to cover up my now destructive emotions and gave me a false sense of courage.

The wild lifestyle continued into my twenties. Now and then, I would get n a bit of trouble. Even though drinking didn't really seem to be that big of a problem, I occasionally stopped. That would only provide fleeting relief. Then once again, a new unexpected health tragedy quickly changed everything.

This time, the vascular surgeons stepped in and told me that I had atherosclerosis, and they would likely have to amputate both my legs. Say what? This was 1986, just before my 28th birthday. After the first two surgeries, I was feeling better, then a few months later, they were ready to cut up my legs again. They told me the arteries had re-blocked and if I didn't have more surgery, I would likely not live very long.

After arguing a bit with the doctors, I refused additional surgery. It just seemed there had to be a better way. Signing out of the hospital against medical advice, I was wheeled to the door and I got out of the chair and started walking with my cane.

I promise that I have a point here. This is the point: Even though I didn't know how I was going to heal, there was still a small loud voice *within* that told me that everything was going to be okay.

This was perhaps one of the first times in my life that I recognized that maybe the answers to life *came from within*. This seemed to work because 35+ years later I'm still here—and today, I do whatever I want. Physically, I'm healthy; I hike up and down mountains, I ski, I ride my bike, and live a pretty darn good life. If you want to learn more about what happened, you'll have to read my first book, "Falling Down Getting UP."

One of the many lessons I've learned along the way is that no matter how sick you are, no matter how messy your life is, you can start over again. The key is to listen *within* and have the guts (yes, sometimes you need a bit of guts) to take massive action. Not a little bit of action, massive immediate action. Or, as I like to say, take a quantum leap!

What I also realized was that 'massive action' didn't have to be complicated. In fact, for me, the simpler the better. In 1987, a doctor at the Pritikin Longevity Center told me to simply get up, walk and don't worry about it. That's right, simply walk and stop worrying. In just two weeks, I went from walking about 10 feet on a cane to walking several miles with a new spring in my step. He told me to eat as much food as I wanted, as long as it was plant-based. And, I started yoga.

I could do that—walking, food, and yoga. *Today, I'm still doing the same three simple things to live a life beyond my wildest imagination.*

Introduction

Part Two
Practices You Can Use

The purpose of this book is to help you realize that you have all the answers you need within you.

Ok, let's get to it. What follows are some ideas you may or may not have thought of—or always thought they wouldn't work for you. My question then is this, "What if it did work for you?" What if the simple tools that are right in front of us, are what can actually help you create a better life?

MINDFULNESS

Mindfulness is the art of being present in the moment and accepting it for what it is. It's a state characterized by awareness, attention, and acceptance without distraction or judgment.

Mindfulness is often used to reduce stress and can lead to greater mental clarity, improved mood, and better physical health. By paying attention to your thoughts, emotions, and sensations, you become less reactive and more responsive, improving relationships and fostering deeper connections.

Mindfulness can also improve the simple pleasures of life by reducing anxiety, depression, and enhancing overall well-being. Whether through meditation or simply being present in daily life, mindfulness can help you achieve greater peace, joy, and connection to the world around you.

Now as long as you're over 16 years old, anyone can practice being mindful. In fact, you're likely doing it already and don't even realize it. Here is how simple it really is.

Have you ever experienced stress while driving? Did you know that you can actually use your time behind the wheel to practice mindfulness?

Mindfulness while driving can be a great way to become more present in the moment and reduce stress and anxiety. One way to practice mindfulness while driving is to focus on your breath. As you inhale and exhale, pay attention to the sensation of air moving in and out of your body. If your mind starts to wander, simply bring your attention back to your breath.

Notice the colors of the cars surrounding you, the signs on the road, and the sounds of the cars and people around you. By focusing on the present moment and the sensory experience, you can become more grounded and less reactive to stress and anxiety.

Finally, you can use your drive time to practice gratitude. Think about the things you are grateful for, such as your health, your family, or your job. By focusing on the positive, you can shift your mindset from one of stress and anxiety to one of gratitude and positivity.

With practice, you can learn to become more mindful in everything you do, simply by driving a car.

BREATHING

Breathing is an essential aspect of life, and it also holds tremendous power when it comes to calming the mind. When we consciously focus on our breath, we can control the pace and rhythm of our breathing, which in turn influences our mental and emotional states.

When I was stressed out for one reason or another as a kid, my mother would simply say, "Michael, take a breath and you'll feel better." It always worked. *Perhaps mothers have this innate intuition and wisdom to know how to breathe in difficult situations.*

Deep, slow breathing can trigger the parasympathetic nervous system, which is responsible for the body's "rest and digest" response. This can lower blood pressure and heart rate, reduce feelings of anxiety, and promote relaxation and calmness.

By focusing on our breath and taking slow, intentional breaths, we can increase oxygen levels in the brain, which can improve cognitive functioning and boost mood. This, in turn, can lead to greater clarity, focus, and mental sharpness.

Breathing can also help us to become more present and grounded in the moment. When we tune in to our breath, we become more aware of our body and surroundings, and less reactive to external stressors. This can help to reduce feelings of overwhelm and improve our ability to respond to challenges in a calm and collected manner.

Simply breathing is another powerful tool for calming the mind and improving overall well-being.

MEDITATION

Meditation is an ancient practice with many benefits for physical, mental and emotional well-being. By using various proven techniques, meditation can reduce stress, lower cortisol levels, and increase relaxation. It can improve mood, reduce symptoms of depression, and increase serotonin levels.

Additionally, meditation can improve physical health by lowering blood pressure, improving respiratory function, reducing chronic pain, and enhancing digestion. It can also improve cognitive function by improving focus, concentration, memory, and decision-making skills.

Certain meditation tools, such as Holosync™, are remarkable science-based tools that can help you go deeper *within*, just by sitting there. There's nothing to do, except put on your headphones and listen to the soothing sounds and music. In a matter of no time at all, you can create a deeper sense of calm and inner peace.

Finally, meditation can have a powerful impact on spiritual well-being, enhancing feelings of purpose and meaning in life. By practicing meditation regularly, it is possible to experience many benefits that can improve your overall quality of life.

Can you believe it?
Simply by sitting calmly for a period of time, you can discover more about your still small voice within.

WALKING

Walking is a simple and accessible form of exercise that has countless benefits for your physical and mental health. One of the primary benefits is that walking is a super low-impact form of exercise, making it easy on the joints and suitable for people of all ages and fitness levels. Walking improves cardiovascular health by increasing heart rate and improving blood flow. This is known to reduce the risk of heart disease, stroke, and other cardiovascular conditions.

In addition to physical health benefits, walking also promotes mental well-being. Research shows that walking can reduce feelings of anxiety and depression, improve mood, and increase overall feelings of well-being. Being out in nature while walking can also reduce stress and improve mental clarity.

Walking regularly can improve cognitive function by boosting memory and concentration. Additionally, walking with others can improve social connections and reduce feelings of loneliness or isolation.

Overall, walking is an easy and effective way to improve physical health, mental well-being, and cognitive function. It can also be a fun and social activity that is suitable for anyone looking to achieve a healthier lifestyle.

By walking only 20 minutes a day, a person takes about 2,000 steps. That's about one mile. If you do that every day, you've walked about 365 miles.

**This simple commitment to walking every day
can change everything.**

NATURE

When it comes to the power of being in nature, there's no denying that it can have a profound effect on the average person. Whether you're hiking off-trail, foraging for mushrooms, or just soaking up some sun by the river, being in nature can wash away all the city energy and leave you feeling at peace.

Not only does nature provide a welcome escape from the hustle and bustle of daily life, but it also has a host of mental and physical health benefits. For instance, studies have shown that spending time in nature can reduce stress levels and improve mood. So, the next time you're feeling overwhelmed by the demands of modern living, consider ditching the concrete jungle for a stroll through the great outdoors.

And let's not forget about the physical benefits of being in nature. Whether you're hiking up a mountain or paddling down a river, spending time in nature often involves physical activity that can improve cardiovascular health, muscle strength, and endurance. Plus, exposure to natural sunlight can help your body produce vitamin D, which is essential for bone health.

**So, if you're feeling stuck in a rut and in need
of a little pick-me-up, take a break from
the screens and get outside.**

YOGA

Yoga combines physical postures, breathing techniques, and meditation to promote overall health and well-being. Its calming effect on the mind and body can reduce tension, stress, and anxiety. Yogic breathing techniques can calm the nervous system, reduce cortisol, and promote relaxation.

Physical postures stretch and release tension promoting flexibility and ease in the body. By cultivating mindfulness, individuals can learn to be present in the moment, reduce anxiety, and achieve a greater sense of awareness and clarity.

Hot Yoga, also known as Bikram Yoga, is a type of Yoga that takes place in a heated and humid environment. Practitioners of Hot Yoga believe it enhances flexibility, detoxification, and cardiovascular health, while also reducing stress levels. The heat can help to relax muscles, increase blood flow, and promote relaxation. Like other forms of Yoga, Hot Yoga combines physical postures, breathing, and meditation. This combination can promote overall health and well-being, enhance focus, and cultivate a greater connection to oneself and the world.

Research shows that Yoga can reduce symptoms of depression and anxiety, improve sleep and mood, and promote better overall health. By incorporating Yoga into daily life, individuals experience lasting and profound benefits for their mental and physical well-being.

Yes, simply by taking time to bend right, bend left, and stretch a bit (especially in a heated room), you can restore your body and mind to their natural working order.

GOING WITHIN

Going *within* is a process of introspection that helps you connect with your deepest desires, values, and beliefs. By exploring your inner world, you gain clarity about what truly matters to you, enabling you to set clear goals and establish intentions leading to an authentic and fulfilling life.

Listening to your still small voice helps provide you with greater clarity and focus, helping you identify the steps needed to achieve your personal goals and overcome limiting beliefs to boost self-confidence. Going *within* fosters self-awareness and mindfulness, which enables you to make conscious choices, builds resilience and emotional intelligence, and galvanizes mental and physical strength to help navigate life's ups and downs.

Incorporating inner work techniques, such as journaling or meditation, to explore your inner world will help you live a life that aligns with your values and aspirations.

Yes, going within can lead you to a more fulfilling life.

NEXT STEP

Mindfulness, breathing, meditation, walking, being in nature, Yoga, and going *within* are all simple, yet powerful practices for helping you to create a truly extraordinary life. You don't even have to do all of them. Start where you are today. Perhaps walk to your local Yoga studio and see what happens.

No pun intended. It's now time to take the next step. What you are about to read in the following 26 revealing essays are incredible personal stories that will have you on the edge of your seat. Each story is unique and offers clues to help you go *within* to live your best life ever.

Who's Michael?

Meet Michael Harris, a multi-talented master of empowering others to succeed. He started practicing yoga in 1987 and was teaching by the early 90's. He's a bestselling author and a personal and business transformation expert. Michael has helped thousands of people share their message with the world and grow their missions. His un-official goal is to hike and ramble up as many buttes as possible, without stumbling down. His even bigger goal is to tell the story of jumping across a deep wide creek on a pogo stick or simply sip a lemonade while watching someone else attempt it first. Of course, all while having fun doing it, and staying at peace *within*.

To learn more about Michael Harris and all the co-authors, visit www.innerpointe.com.

To go *within*, simply turn the page.

The Essays
Within

"Before embarking on important undertakings
sit quietly, calm your senses and thoughts,
& meditate deeply. You will then be guided
by the great creative power of Spirit."

~ Paramahansa Yogananda

Michele Vennard

Essay One

"Living From Grief"

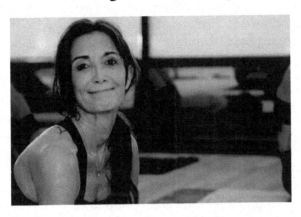

Even as I sit here writing, ready to pour my passionate words on paper about this yoga that I believe in, I'm incredibly sad.

My sister sits next to me coloring. She's visiting as she does each year for six weeks after having been diagnosed with early-onset Alzheimer's...

...the very reason why I started yoga in the first place as my mom also had this devastating condition, passing 25 years ago at age 54.

My sister and I have ALWAYS been close, even at young ages when kids are supposed to have sibling rivalry. Not us. We had many of the same friends and while different—she likes tea, I like coffee—we are as close today as we were then.

My Mom was in that pack too, so losing her was traumatic to both my sister and me.

Like a frog in water, I didn't realize the stress building in me throughout my entire life in every situation: a neglected relationship, a work-obsessed schedule, digestive IBS problems, and a simple lack of feeling any joy.

I'd often think, "How can I be happy? My mom is dying."

Mom passed away on March 2nd, 1998. It wasn't pretty, and yet having her pass in my arms awakened a feeling of wanting to live life like I hadn't before. A strange mix of emotions ensues when life ends; I felt mad, sad, confused, and abandoned but also less anxious, ready for change, courageous, and daring.

But, in that time, many other things became less important. Even though I loved my work, the meaning behind it began to fade. I was less social and didn't want to engage in what I thought were "silly" conversations. I bought books on angels, began to write prose, and developed a card line with my original photos coming from my grandfather's camera. I was pretty nutty and unrelatable in normal ways and I knew it.

Why? What's the point anyway?

Pretty cynical sounding but really, as I see it now, a new version of myself was blossoming. I'm a hugely determined human being so it's going to take something fairly relentless to get me to listen AND change course. I had several appointments at that time with a Stanford Gastroenterologist as my digestion, swelling, and constipation were impossible to deal with. It was embarrassing, depressing, and very painful.

On a flight home from Denver, looking through an inflight magazine, I caught a glimpse of a person in a Yoga pose. I recalled some friends of mine telling me to try Yoga to help me cope with this monumental list of emotions and behaviors that had me unidentifiable.

There wasn't anything specific that I read. I just had a feeling of "Why not?"

Waking up one morning, eyes to the ceiling in grief, I decided that was it. Grabbing the phone book, I scanned down to see a yoga studio on Filbert Street. I drove down the street and perfectly timed my arrival for class, walked in stating, "I'm the one that called, brand new to any Yoga."

Reading the San Francisco Chronicle, this elegant man stood up and told me with his thick accent what to fill out, what the payment was, and where to go and wait. I walked into this small room that had black flooring and mirrors and noticed people laying down on mats. It was super strange, but I pretended to know what I was doing and found a corner that I thought could hide my insecurities and presence.

The teacher, Tony, came in, turned the lights on, and we stood while he proceeded to give instructions on how to do things with our bodies. I was intimidated, completely uncoordinated, mentally disoriented, and with my body screaming, I knew I was *in the right place for sure*. At one point, I couldn't hold back the tears and just let them flow with my heart hyperventilating in me.

I knew then it was the release that I needed and not the unceasing amount of control I was creating that could help the wacky state that I was in.

I laid there after class, in my own lovely toil and with a lightness of being.

I knew that I'd be doing this again and again. And, I did.

I noticed clearly how I started to feel.

I noticed an extra skip in my step.

I felt connected to the world.

Despite the unknown of where I was going in my life, my stomach problems were feeling better. I managed my feelings without losing myself in them. It's like the papers spilled out all over the floor were suddenly swept up and placed neatly back into their proper files, sorted and useful.

Still, in my career of opening restaurants, I inquired about where to go to take this yoga in other areas of the west coast. Tony shared with me, "Anywhere you see a Bikram's College of India" you are fine. Politely, I said, "Thank you" but wondered if he misunderstood me. Bikram College of India, what is that?

Walking into a Yoga studio in Kirkland, Washington, I instantly felt the heat and noticed a poster of my teacher hanging up on his wall in the reception area. "Hi, I'm Michele, visiting here from California." Getting through all the formalities of paperwork, purchase, and etiquette, I asked, "Why do you have a poster of my teacher on your wall?" He said only, "Your teacher is Tony?" and walked away to do his other duties.

What happened in that room was a joke.

First of all, I could barely see as the steam was so thick. Secondly, I don't remember what I did as I sat a lot and was in complete shock at the amount of sweat that I could produce. The cab driver who picked me up stared at me as I approached his car, and asked, "Are you okay, what happened?" Hooked, I made an arrangement with that cab driver to pick me up each day at 7 a.m. to take a Yoga class while I was here to open restaurants.

Funny how life hits you. I continued to live in various worlds, having duties in restaurants, some in the card business, and some as a concierge. I was still running, doing more Yoga, and in a new relationship, all to heal and grow.

I believe now this was a "hallway" in my life, with doors closing and new ones opening.

It's a tough place to be in but necessary as the insights coming from those moments are key ingredients to a vision that in due course will reveal itself to you. For me, what started to grow in the midst of all this was the indescribable and unmistakable benefit this yoga was giving to countless people.

Now going to Global Yoga headed by Mary, the lines of people eagerly waiting to get in and fit in rooms no larger than 700-900 square feet. Not one person minded being mat to mat, feet to nose; you could be heavy, thin, old, young, shiny and new, wrinkled and bent over. No color, language, hair, or no hair, mattered. Where you lived, what you did, or the car you drove was absolutely irrelevant.

It was inclusive. You were here for a reason not unlike mine; something stirred in you enough and you were going to take care of it right here. In so doing, we were one. Those times baffled me and reminded me of my mom. She knew no difference between a toll collector and a pastor at church; she gave you the time of day.

Yoga helped me be seen in my misery and it was helping others be seen in theirs.

While heading to a family reunion in New York—I was leaving my restaurant life, though still doing work as a concierge but now full-on developing a card catalog with my original photos and prose to sell in hospital shops and boutiques, with portions of proceeds going to hospice—I reclined back in my seat to read a pamphlet about a yoga seminar that maybe I'd attend. Going through it a bit more clearly, I saw that it was for Teacher Training. I shook my head and said to myself, "Oh I misunderstood what this was," and put it back under the chair.

As you might guess, above the clouds without my normal task list, I thought only about what it would be like to be a teacher. By the time we landed, I was going and KNEW God helped me knit together all the pieces you've kindly just taken the time to read, leading me into this glorious life of teaching and owning a studio for over 20 years!

Fast forward to today...

I'd be lying if I didn't say how upset I am that I have to live through another experience of dementia with the very person I've done my whole life with, my sister. Truth is, that's a selfish comment and I know it.

The good news is that yoga has taught me to go within, to live more because of the grief, and to do so with more patience than I had with my mom.

Here's another truth: we are all going to die. Sounds grim but again, Yoga taught me to KNOW that with loving awareness. It's freeing, actually, because each moment IS precious; each moment IS new, and each moment counts. I can navigate a broken heart better than I did before.

While still painful to have lost my mom, I now know how to take care of myself AND be present and LIVE in the time I do have with people that I love, and serve this and any situation in a loving exemplary manner

My 3 Tips for You...

1. Trust the process. You will grow in faith in yourself and God.

2. Think longevity. Keep your perspective on the long game, this will take the pressure off; this is a marathon, not a sprint. Don't expect to grow in a straight line. It will get messy but you're still moving forward.

3. If you make this the foundation for your life—the cornerstone, the one rock all others count on—all else will fall into place.

Who's Michele?

Michele Vennard's closet wall is covered with meaningful photos and messages that she's collected over the years from many students. "It validates what I am doing with my life's purpose and that feels good." As the Founder and owner of Bikram Yoga San Jose, established in 2003, she received her Bikram's Teacher certificate in 2001. Michele has participated in Yoga competitions around the world and won the women's divisions in the U.S. National and the India International Yoga Competitions.

To learn more about Michele Vennard and all the co-authors, visit www.innerpointe.com.

Dr. Avi Sharma

Essay Two

"Improving your health—keep it simple."

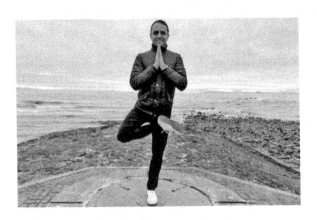

No-one truly knows you better than you know yourself. This *qualifies* you to be able to take some initial, safe steps to optimize your own health. Most of us have experienced the challenges of starting, and certainly maintaining, a new habit. That's why these initial steps need to be simple and easily accessible for you.

At 24 years old, I had my first significant injury to my right knee. The Orthopedic Surgeon said,

"You're a doctor, not a professional footballer... stop playing football!"

Tough to hear, as back then football was my main release; it was where I felt most free and was able to catch up with my brother and some of my closest friends.

However, by continuing to play there was a chance the cartilage tears and the early osteoarthritic changes could both get worse, potentially requiring a knee replacement in my 50s!

Weighing these risks against the huge benefits I got from continuing to play football, and by taking that accountability, I was a happier individual for it. I was living my best life, or I would 'die by my own sword,' with no-one to blame, especially not my surgeon—who was fantastic by the way.

It's ironic, a healthcare professional not taking the advice of another healthcare professional, and now asking you to listen to my story. There's a difference, though; I'm not asking you to listen *to me,* but rather for you to hopefully listen *to yourself.* As healthcare professionals, teachers, or anyone who influences another person's health or situation, we should try to *better listen* to what the human being in front of us ideally wants to happen. No-one likes being told what to do, but if the treatment plan or suggestion is a *joint decision* then it's more likely to be implemented.

Turns out my Orthopedic Surgeon was right though—things got worse!

Despite efforts of rehabilitation through physiotherapy, continuing to play the beautiful game was *wrecking* my knee. At times, I struggled to walk even fifty yards without excruciating pain.

My wife and I love to walk. On holiday, we enjoy nothing more than walking two hours for a coffee just chatting, being together, and enjoying the sun. Stopping every 10 minutes wasn't really adding to the experience!

At 28 years old, I had knee surgery, where they shaved away some of the torn cartilage. Despite the correct pre- and post-operation physiotherapy, my knee just never felt the same. As years passed, my knee felt weak and kept giving way; my next injury always felt like it was just around the corner.

By 34 years old, I decided something needed to change, especially as the expert advice was now once again for knee surgery.

Looking into who played football for the longest, Ryan Gigg's name kept coming up. He's often spoken of the contribution yoga made to extending his career at Manchester United, helping him play at the highest level into his early 40s. So, I researched and found my local Bikram Yoga Studio in Glasgow, taking my first class in April 2014. I fell in love with the practice immediately, feeling fresher, lighter, and stronger. The combination of this 90-minute hot yoga session once a week, and strength training, over a six-month period completely transformed my knee problems—I became **pain-free.**

I canceled my planned second knee surgery and I have never looked back!

I'm so glad to have returned to enjoying our long family walks in the sun. One of my current issues is that while I can play football with no knee concerns, and can run harder and faster than I could in my 20s, I now struggle to find enough time to play!

I guess we are all a work in progress.

The experience with my knee, and the *side effect* of **feeling more in control** of my general life pressures, led me to dive deeper into the incredible healing potential of yoga.

For the past seven years, I've had two main working roles as a General Practitioner (GP/ Family Doctor) and a Yoga Teacher, having completed my teacher training in Thailand, in November 2016. I'm hugely passionate about each of these roles, and love them both equally.

Improving our health can feel so complicated with all the *information overload* out there, so let's try keeping it simple...

Your body is **designed to move;** the more you move, the better you will feel[1]. As little as 10 minutes of regular light activity, like **walking,** can affect the electrical activity and structures of emotional processing areas of your brain[2]. If you struggle to walk, then move your arms or your legs, or intermittently just brace your core[3]. *Any* movement counts in a positive way!

By attending an **activity class that you enjoy,** you will have fun developing a skill, being part of a community, feeling connected, and sharing the purpose of reaching an end goal.

Yoga offers additional benefits by teaching you how to stay present. You learn how to have better control of your breath, body, and mind. This develops and builds on your inherent resilience both in the class, yet more importantly outside the class.

A further chapter is really required to do justice to the evidence behind the benefits that yoga offers. These include reducing inflammation within the body, improving balance within the nervous system, increasing chemical messengers within the brain that exert a calming effect, supporting positive brain changes (neuroplasticity), and gaining better control over your thought processes[4].

Most yoga classes have a foundation on **breath control.** On average, we breathe 25,000 breaths per day, but how many of these do we *consciously* think about? As a population, we tend to breathe too fast and too often[5]. **Nasal breathing** is our most efficient way to breathe—in through the nose, and out through the nose. **

Practice is key, so let's give it a go:

• Breathe in (inhale) for 3-5 seconds, and then breathe out (exhale) for 3-5 seconds, both through your nose.

- With each round try to breathe slower, fuller, but also *lighter* - aiming to find a comfortable, soft rhythm.

- Continue this **intentional nasal breathing** for 2 minutes – also, try softening your gaze or even closing your eyes.

- Please take a genuine moment to **notice how you feel** after this.

The better you become at nasal breathing, the more efficiently you deliver oxygen to your lungs and the more energy you will have, for less effort[5]. Breathing through your nose also filtrates and humidifies air, acting as a first line of defense for your airways and leading to less moisture loss.

Learning to improve your breathing is free, available to everyone, and can be performed *anywhere,* even while watching Netflix or walking in the park.

Over time, making it a habit to be **more aware of your breathing** will help you become a *less reactive* person, with the potential to positively impact *any* relationship you have—imagine that!

Master this breathing technique and you will be a less stressed, more resilient individual with more self-awareness for any challenges you face. Rather than just accepting *what is happening to me,* you will focus more on *what I can do to help my situation.*

There has never been a better time to safely learn how to have more ownership of our health and well-being, given the huge pressures facing all our healthcare services.

Improving different areas of our **lifestyle**—*breathing, sleep, movement, nutrition, light exposure, relaxation, kindness, connection/ relationships, meaning/ purpose, and avoidance of substance abuse/ addiction*—can each complement modern medicine to help make significant positive changes to our overall health.

However, by simply **starting to be more conscious and more aware of your breathing,** even a little more than you currently do - through movement practices like yoga - can slowly start to improve each of those lifestyle areas mentioned above.

I really hope you can relate, in some way, to the significant impact yoga has had on each of the wonderful people in this book, who may even have faced similar challenges to you.

At 43 years old, I'm a happier, stronger person who reacts more calml (*most* of the time!) to the many curveballs that life will throw at us. I'm ver proud to be married to my soulmate, and together we have created ou wee miracle baby daughter, who defied logic to come into this world. I fee so grateful and blessed for the family, friends, and worldwide connection in our life. I also believe it's no coincidence that so much of this fulfillmen has occurred since I took my first hot yoga class in 2014.

The highest recommendation I can give to yoga is this...

My wife and I have no interest in pushing our daughter into anything we just hope she is happy, follows her passions, and that she lives her life as a kind and compassionate individual. However, she will absolutely be encouraged to adopt a yoga practice as I believe this will create a positive impact in *all areas of her life*—from challenges she may face to goals she hopes to achieve. She will be able to listen to her own body and mind better, *from within*, allowing for more clarity and purpose in whicheve path(s) she chooses.

Yoga will allow our baby girl to love herself more, and to better share love with those whom she cares for.

My 3 Tips for You...

1. **Intentional breathing.** *Slowing down* in life is something we all need to work on, particularly with our *breathing*. Commit to practicing two minutes of uninterrupted intentional nasal breathing, every day.

2. **Move more.** Find a movement practice that you enjoy and commit to a regular weekly practice.

3. **Be patient.** People often give up on health interventions because they don't see results within a few days or weeks. Most of us have been drawn into the '6-week program' of something. Start by shifting this approach to make small changes which *you can sustain* for 6 months, 6 years, or even 6 decades!

Who's Avi?

Dr. Avi Sharma is a General Practitioner (Family Doctor/ GP) and Yoga Teacher with a passion for breath, movement, and lifestyle medicine. He hopes to help empower people to make small, safe, and sustainable changes to aspects of their lifestyle, which in turn have long-term positive impacts on their overall health and emotional well-being.

To learn more about Dr. Avi Sharma and all the co-authors, visit www.innerpointe.com.

** If struggling with nasal polyps or chronic nasal congestion, please initially speak with your healthcare provider.

*References 1,2,3,4,5. Please see "References and Citations" in the back of the book

Eddie & Emily Garner

Essay Three

"Practice:
How Doing the Same Thing
is Never the Same"

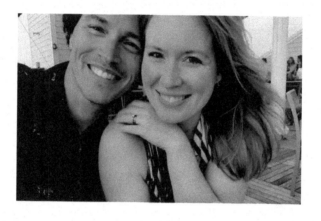

Supposedly, Albert Einstein once said, "Insanity is doing the same thing over and over and expecting different results."

Urban legend or not, it's a great quote. Interestingly enough, this is exactly what we do when we practice a Yoga posture. We try, try again with the hope that something will be better—and, with enough practice, it will indeed be better. The reason this repeated practice is not insanity is that someone else has already done the work for us. Thousands of years ago, the technique of Yoga practice was created to provide the body with the greatest therapeutic benefit and the least amount of negative impact. Yoga itself is not the goal; our ever-changing bodies and minds are. The technique remains the same, and we just get to do our best in any given moment and try the technique again, each time for the first time.

It is never actually the same.

We both came from backgrounds in opera and ballet. In those classical art forms, technique dominates. (One could argue that any consistently successful person has some sort of structural technique they live by). The artist strives to develop an approach that will allow them to duplicate work accurately and on demand, and from year to year. Although the attention to technique may stem solely from a selfish desire to be able to present a skill or material confidently, the artist will usually discover that...

...the technique begets freedom.

Rather than listening to an often-harsh inner voice, the artist can focus on an approach that has consistently worked for them in the past, achieve desired results, and then get to focus on the fun part—the making of their art. In a sense, the artist walks an ever-shifting line between real-time self-observation (to have consistent technique) and the spontaneity and/or desire of the present moment. Having a ground floor of consistent technique is really the only way you can even come close to guaranteeing results.

This is equally true of practicing Yoga. If a student only strives to look a certain way in a posture, then they risk being disappointed most days. Our bodies are constantly helping us cope with physical and mental stressors. With stress levels so varied, how could we expect our bodies, or our minds, for that matter, to perform the same from day to day?

Technique frees us from the burden of judgment, the feeling of disappointment in progress, and the "why haven't I gotten there yet?" If we know exactly what muscles we are to contract and basically what the ideal positioning of the body for therapeutic benefit is, we can confidently move forward without the feeling of defeat on our bad days.

Any technique involves discipline, and discipline informs the choices we make on our bad days.

That constant practice creates a cumulative result, and in mastering the technique, something else can be created. The technique is not the result. Practicing and then learning the technique allows for **something to be created** from it. The dancer must practice and master basic movements. Those basic movements are not the dance—they allow for the dance to happen. The singer must practice and master basic vocal skills. Those sounds are not the music—they allow for the music to happen. The yogi, too, practices basic skills (asana, breath control, stillness). Those basics are not the totality of Yoga. Those basics allow Yoga to happen. **And what you've created is your life.**

Over the past 18 years, we have had the great pleasure of teaching the solid technique of Bikram Yoga, not just to lots of students, but also to many consistent students over that entire time frame. Right before our eyes, we have watched miraculous transformations occur in people who often had no idea they needed to change. They were distracting themselves with all sorts of things in an effort to mask the feeling of something just not being right. They tried Yoga because maybe some pictures on social media or some celebrity story made them think they should. Yet, they later realized they were being called towards it by their own desire to embrace their inner being.

Eddie: It was obvious to me from my first class that Yoga was the only thing I had ever done truly for myself. The instructions come at you with such honesty that they force you to take ownership of your body and the way it moves. You are so eager to listen because you know immediately that it's for your own good. If you learn nothing else from Yoga, you learn that no one is going to do it for you. In any given class, you have students ranging from experts in their field to the occupationally lost. You may have students who are very wealthy sweating next to someone who is barely making it financially. This hodgepodge of humanity came to the class for different reasons, and yet all for the same thing—themselves.

Emily: I went to class on a whim. I loved it immediately, but at first, I struggled because my type-A mind wanted to perform—kick the highest and balance the longest. So, I suffered, but still, I loved it. And then maybe a month in, my teacher said to me, "We all know you're flexible. When are you going to start practicing yoga?" And man, all of a sudden, I didn't have to perform; I could change my focus from outward to inward, and the world opened up.

"Yoga is the first time you fall in love with yourself because it is the first time you actually see yourself." – **Bikram Choudhury**

When you have a group of people so diverse, you must have a very specific approach to your instruction. At any given moment, the star athlete and the couch potato both need to know exactly what to do. With our background in the arts, we were just so used to self-observation and attention to detail. Of course, we were drawn to how specific Bikram Yoga is. And yet, where we, like so many artists (or people in general), had habits of toxic self-talk and judgment about the many ways we weren't good enough, this new technique provided the opposite. Any attempt was indeed good enough, and with honest effort and attention to this technique, it was obvious that it was working. It was total freedom. We wanted so badly to share this freedom with others.

Getting students and keeping students are two different things.

A student in their thirties may only be coming to Yoga to burn calories. A student in their seventies may only be coming to still feel part of a community after retirement and/or the loss of a spouse. These are equally valuable reasons.

How can one class make both of these people happy?

Because everything is relative. And the moment you stop comparing yourself to something else, and instead do the work you know you need for YOU in any given moment, doors start opening.

This idea of keeping students believing in their own progress is one of the hardest things about teaching. (Doesn't that sound silly? We all would tell **someone else** they should believe in themself, but somehow, belief in one's own self is one of the most difficult things any given person can accomplish). How can you convince the student whose belly is keeping them from touching their forehead to their knee that they'll get there eventually? How do you keep someone with chronic back pain believing that relief could be only a few classes (or even a few postures) away? The answer is undoubtedly different for everyone. What has worked for us is to keep the students interested in the technique of the postures. "Trying the right way and receiving 100% of the therapeutic benefit" has been a mantra. We do our best to keep our students only "judging" (that is, noticing) the attention with which they are attempting the instructions (that is, the technique), rather than what they look like or how deeply they are going into the postures.

We have taught some of the same students through three decades of their lives. Maybe they started in their thirties and are now in their fifties. Or maybe they started in their fifties and are now in their seventies. To be perfectly honest, many of them haven't aged a day. They are in many ways more vibrant than they were when we met them. We've watched them crawl around on the floor with the same grandchildren (and great-grandchildren) that are now about to head to college. All the while, taking the same yoga class, with the same technique, and with many of the same people. In a phase of life where one may feel things are ending, we see Yoga students feel like they are just getting started. The continuity of the class has been a stronghold for so many of us. Our reason for practicing is always slightly different, but somehow, Yoga knows exactly why we are there.

Sweet, peaceful relief is always *within you,* and the beginning is only one breath, one class away.

Our 3 Tips for You...

1. You are the most interesting thing in everything you do. Be confident in your selfishness while you practice Yoga. Look for the little details that make an enormous difference.

2. No Yoga posture is worth you losing your inner sense of peace, and the only thing that can take away your inner peace is holding your breath. Redemption is only ever one breath away.

3. Celebrate every little success. The only person who needs to believe in you is YOU.

Who are Eddie & Emily?

Eddie & Emily Garner excel at restoring hope to people who are not sure where to begin to get their lives back. Since 2005, their main focus has been specializing in teaching Yoga to students with major physical challenges, professional athletes, and everything in between. Together, their goal is to promote health and happiness through Yoga.

To learn more about Eddie & Emily Garner and all the co-authors, visit www.innerpointe.com.

Gretchen Olsen

Essay Four

"The Observer"

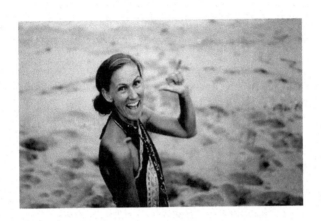

Humans are fascinating.

Watching (and learning) from them is one of my favorite pastimes.

My life is like a sitcom episode.

Truly.

It's hilarious!!

As a kid, I was very quiet and shy. Most of the things I really wanted to learn, I spent much time observing before I tried. Ice skating, horse riding, volleyball, cooking, driving a stick shift, AND the most rewarding one, being a mom. Perfectionist? Maybe. Afraid to mess up? You bet! A flight attendant for 20 years, a Bikram Yoga student, teacher and studio owner, and best for last... a MOM for 15 years!! Shout out to all the mamas out there!! You are so epic!! I love to laugh, so that helps.

How does this relate to Yoga you ask? Read on...

There is something about seeking truth, YOUR truth, at your own pace. I have a note behind the front desk at my studio that says...

"Truth will correct ALL errors in my mind."

My truth may not be yours but one great thing about being an observer is that you can take what is useful for you and leave the rest!

You are always a choice.

Master Kuthumi says, "Knowledge is learned, and wisdom is remembered."

Are you aware of the wisdom that is *within* you? It's in there!

Sometimes we resist and of course, then we struggle. Confession: I am definitely resisting writing this, and I know I want and need to do this!

Resistance in Yoga class is very common. The posture we think we are the worst at is of course the one we need the most. Hint: You are never "bad" at Yoga postures if you listen and try the correct way. In fact, be excited about the ones you can't do—yet. They are helping you the most!

We, humans, are very funny. For most people, it seems the hardest Yoga posture is just showing up.

Yup, did you know when you show up for the most important person in your life (Psst...that is YOU) how much better the world is as a result?

Seems small but through over 15 years of standing on my observation deck (my Yoga mat, and the podium, teaching) I can clearly see how much each of us is affecting EV-ERY-THING! Not to mention all of the wonderful stories I get to hear about the lives of my students outside of the studio.

YOU ARE AMAZING! Just thought I'd let you know.

Because it is just for me, I love my Yoga practice. Every physical activity I had done in my life before Yoga was competitive. I loved those as well, and they did serve a purpose at the time, but I really love the freedom and zero pressure from my Yoga practice today.

In my early years of Yoga, I had so many stops and starts. Excuses were abundant. Mostly the cost of the class, but of course, the time it required. How can I fly away from my child for two or three days and then justify going to Yoga when I am finally home with him?

My sister, Shannon, and I are both certified Bikram Yoga teachers. Our poor parents; they are both over 70 and practice regularly. No choice? *They* should be writing a chapter in this book! They inspire me every day to keep trying to get pure Bikram Yoga out to as many people as possible. Shan and I attended our first yoga class in 2005 at Bikram Yoga Fremont Street in Portland, OR. Shout out to Michael Harris for starting this amazing healing space back in 1999!

Who knew that 11 years later, I would become co-owner of the studio with my friend Danelle?! Both Shan and I had been practicing various forms of Hatha yoga prior to our Bikram Yoga and were definitely a bit "judgy" about the goings-on at the studio. It seemed like a weird (and stinky!) place to do Yoga. After buying the cheap deal for a month of Yoga, we headed into the class where we continued our questioning of this establishment.

We both had the same thoughts...

That's not Tree Pose! That's definitely not Triangle Posture!

And above all, WHY *did we wear these long pants in such a hot room!?*

But we listened and tried and struggled and... WOW!! Sorry, no questions asked. None. I will always remember our bike ride home from that first class. That will certainly be one of my life's sitcom episodes.

The favorite person I like to observe is this amazing 15-year-old who I am lucky enough to call my son. I hope he allows me to put him in this chapter because he is always my inspiration. When we brought him home from the hospital on day three of his life, I was blown away that they let us take him home! How could we be trusted with this perfect specimen? It was the most nerve-racking four-mile drive of my life! When Vaughn was two years old, I had many questions. How do I get him to do what I want him to do!? Ha! Why does he not listen to me and do as I say all the time?

One day, it really hit me how much of an observer my son was, and that he was always watching me. Not just watching, but feeling my emotions and expressing them to me.

My son was my own little mirror.

If I want my child, or anyone for that matter, to do something, then I had better be fully prepared to do it myself. To be honest, I was very distraught over this new realization.

Do you ever get distraught over your realizations?

Gulp! Does this mean I have to be perfect all the time? When I called my dad, he gave me the ole "Yep, sorry to break it to ya kid!"

Even though I've tried many other therapies, nothing on the planet does what Bikram Yoga does for me. Since I know I need to be there, I stand on my observation deck (mat) most days of the week. As I write this, we are currently at the end of a 28-day Self-Love Challenge at my studio here in Kapaa, Kauai. Teaching most of the classes each month, somehow, I still manage to get my practice in almost daily. All the students help me to hold myself accountable. They are also my mirrors and super supporters. Shout out to the BYK family!

If I don't dedicate myself to my practice, I've neglected the most important person in my life—Me.

Who's the most important person in your life?

Luck sets in! After my one-month yoga intro ended, I stopped my practice because I thought I couldn't afford it. How is that lucky, you might ask? I took the winter off from yoga during my first winter in Portland. Umm… Ya, I know, stay with me here and trust the process.

I got married on January 1, 2006, then on my birthday in March, I got gift certificates to go back to the hot sweaty studio on Fremont Street.

Ding! Ding! Ding!

Both my mom and husband knew what I wanted and needed. I went back to yoga and quickly used up my gift. Then, by the grace of the Gods and Goddesses, I was able to get in on a three-month summer special that cheap ole me felt was justifiable.

Apparently, Portlandians don't like to do hot Yoga in the summer.

Whaaaaaat?

Committing to my Bikram Yoga practice, I began skipping my runs even though I was training for a race. Actually, I ended up with my best race time ever by practicing Yoga more rather than taking training runs.

At the peak of my health, I became pregnant with my one and only Vaughn. Being new to the practice, someone told me that I shouldn't do hot Yoga while pregnant. Good news, I actually listened to that person.

Trust the process.

Instead, I went back to my running, walking, and at-home pregnancy Yoga with no heat. Bummer. Another chance to prove myself, right? I wanted so much to be in the hot room! I needed the sweat so very much and didn't listen to ME.

Today, my mission is to support EVERY student to start *and* continue their yoga practice, especially during a journey to motherhood. It is a time of strength in a woman's life and in fact, it is the time in your life when you are most tuned into your body and your baby's body as it grows inside of you! You definitely must be an "observer" when you are carrying another human inside you. Often, I say that everyone should practice as if they are pregnant!

Don't most moms advocate more for their children, than they do for themselves?

Not saying that it's right, but through my observations, it is mostly the truth. Where we may not stand up for ourselves, we will always go to bat for our kids. Now, to apply that to ME, the most important person in my life. Put my mask (oxygen) on first before assisting anyone else. There is no other way. As a flight attendant, I don't know how many moms I have told to put their masks on first, before helping their babies. It is a hard concept to embrace.

My questions for you...

Are you *really* listening? Are you observing your life? Are you going WITHIN?

My 3 Tips for You...

1. Never, EVER, give up!

2. Be your BIGGEST fan and cheerleader!

3. Be BRAVE and come visit me in Kauai!

Who's Gretchen?

Gretchen Olsen is a mom, yoga teacher and small business owner who lives in Hawaii. She loves the ocean and Yoga, so the islands are a perfect spot to live. Since 2019, she has led a strong little Yoga hale in Kapaa, called Bikram Yoga Kauai. Gretchen loves sharing with anyone and everyone what is possible through a consistent and dedicated practice.

To learn more about Gretchen Olsen and all the co-authors, visit www.innerpointe.com.

Rowena Jayne

Essay Five

"Sometimes You Have to Lose Yourself To Find Yourself Again."

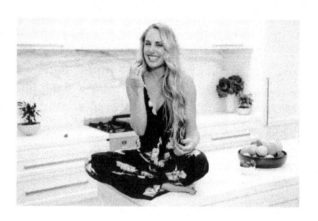

It's 6 a.m. and a new day.

A golden hue envelops the room as the warm sun penetrates the glass of the window. This is a recurring moment I have come to relish as I flip my Yoga mat in the air and watch it unravel and land on the floor. Heater on, mouth closed, eyes open...

My daily, non-negotiable Yoga practice begins.

My practice is and has been my lifeline; my go-to; the way I begin my day.

Moments on the mat are sacred and I cherish the myriad of explorative and insightful journeys *within* it has gifted me as a reward for my dedication and twenty-year commitment to this time-honored "spiritual" practice.

Yoga is first and foremost my teacher, however, since its first inception into my life it also poses as my ally, my friend, and my guide.

Yoga has been an underlying catalyst in creating a diverse level of success in my life. I have my own successful service-based business in the health and wellness space; I have great relationships and have achieved many accolades, awards, and significance-based success. However, my greatest chievement is the vibrancy, joy, passion, and confidence I have cultivated hrough Yoga. The best part is: **I live a heart-centered, enriched life.**

However, it wasn't always this way...

Desperate to change my life, in 2003, I lay on a cold hospital bed, having been admitted with a bleeding colon. Before being hospitalized, I struggled with Rheumatoid Arthritis (RA) and an eating disorder.

The eating disorder seemingly called the shots. Over ten years, I had shoved chocolate, chips, and other crunchy, salty, sugary processed foods into my mouth to suppress the pain, fear, hurt, anger, sadness, and injustice of my life. Struggling with weight, body image, emotional eating, and starving, my metabolism was debilitated, and I basically and ruthlessly hated myself.

In our youth, it's difficult to distinguish whether the family we are born into is dysfunctional. In hindsight, clearly, mine was. My birth father was a violent, abusive alcoholic with a Bipolar diagnosis. Growing up, home life was a turbulent wave of fear and uncertainty, while lacking any grounded resources to offer a sense of safety.

My father stumbled home drunk one night and instigated a fight with my mother. She hastily relocated my sisters and me to the kitchen, directing us to eat dinner while she dealt with his rage. Though not an eyewitness to events, the pleading, screams, and loud thumps as he kicked her down the stairs were piercingly distinguishable while I scoffed my dinner as instructed to avoid my own mayhem. I understand this moment was a pivotal juncture in the onset of my eating disorder. The trigger: When life is stressful, dangerous, or under threat, eat.

Human beings are extremely adaptable and resilient; we always find ways to weather life's storms. I grew up always trying to be a good girl and people-pleasing to avoid pain. I pushed myself to be the best at everything in an attempt to be untouchable and feel worthy. However, human conditioning known as repetition compulsion ensured I continuously repeated the same or similar situations of abuse over and over in my life.

I aspired to create a "high life" for myself.

I was always chasing the highs to avoid the lows. My passion for the theater led me to complete a performing arts and acting degree, allowing me to travel the world performing on stage and screen.

At 25, I met my husband while performing in Singapore, which stirred up unresolved pain around men and provoked me to contact my birth father.

This decision was the catalyst for a long stint of abuse and death threats. I would receive my father's drunken, abusive, and threatening phone calls sometimes up to 13 times a day. The abuse eventually scared me to the point of acquiring a domestic violence order to protect myself.

The trauma and stress took its toll on my immune system, leaving me with Rheumatoid Arthritis in my left knee. The swelling was horrendous and I wasn't able to walk. The doctor's prognosis suggested I'd never heal, that rheumatoid factor and high CRP would be prevalent in my blood for life, and my only solution was a life sentence of anti-inflammatories. I refused.

With frankness, the hospital doctor spoke: "We think you have Crohn's disease, an aggressive, inflammatory bowel disease." My mind began to spin, yet simultaneously I heard another voice whispering to me in response:

"You don't have Crohn's; this is your wake-up call to change your life or stay on the same trajectory and destroy it".

I couldn't decipher the words' origin but they were irrefutable and brought forth a sense of hope. I knew deep in my heart I needed to listen and adhere to this voice.

Upon hospital discharge, I sought solace in prayer. I truly believe all prayers are answered if we ask for what we want with clarity and intention. I hobbled along the street with my rickety, swollen, arthritic knee and someone called my name. I looked around, only to be met with silence and no visual that matched the audible words.

Then it came—the same voice from the hospital:

"Look up."

I raised my head and tilted my eyes toward the sky to see what felt like an intervention leading to a new chapter and a new way of experiencing life. The answer to my prayer was a simple sign flapping in the breeze; it read: "Bikram Yoga Lane Cove, Grand Opening." To me, it was glaringly obvious and provided no scope for contention.

Scurrying to the door, I grabbed the timetable, and in an hour, I was in my first class. I struggled to execute the postures with my swollen, painful knee and avoided eye contact with myself in the mirror.

Nonetheless, I felt more alive and energized than ever before.

A distinct change arose after my first class—I came home with healthy food cravings and despite all my adversity, within one month of practicing 4-5 times a week, the pain and swelling were all but gone from my knee. My dietary habits changed dramatically; I lost weight, toned my body, and my disposition improved tremendously, generating happiness and contentment *within*. I also no longer have a rheumatoid factor or elevated CRP in my blood.

In just three Yoga classes, I knew *within*, I was destined to become a teacher and was certified at an in-depth training in 2005.

On day one of training, the "Om Song" was played. I lay in Savasana, tears streaming down my cheeks as the lyrics boomed from the loudspeaker:

"Hey you, looking for life. You need look no further, it's here. Peace may be found here in your heart. You hold the key, Yoga is life."

The seeker in me had searched high and low to heal my life. I had been lost though I knew in my heart I was now at the crossroad out of the darkness, into the light. I was on the path of self-discovery where "yoga makes you, *you*."

Yoga became the underpinning of healing my life in a psycho-spiritual, psychosomatic way. One class, as I dived deeply into camel pose, a thought entered my mind:

"If my own father doesn't love me, why would anyone else?"

Sobbing profusely for the entirety of the class, the teacher intuitively sat beside me and invited me to roar like a lion. As I followed his advice, emotion erupted and transformed into total empowerment. It felt so good that I repeated the roar and to my surprise, the entire class of 199 students joined in with me! That moment taught me Yoga is the catalyst for purging deep physical and emotional pain.

Yoga can enable you to cultivate an ever-evolving door into your heart, mind, and soul to witness where you are on any given day.

Throughout all the years of my practice, I have purged, laughed, cried, and screamed. It's been a safe haven to explore the varied kaleidoscope of pent-up emotions and feelings associated with my trauma, alongside the inner and outer relationships I have with my identity, life, and others.

Children growing up in traumatic environments often experience hypervigilance—existing on high alert in an attempt to adapt to the lack of safety and certainty. [1] Yoga provides a valuable resource for regulating the nervous system and offering a sense of safety where there once was not.

It is well-recognized that stress and/or trauma create dysregulation of the neuroendocrine, immune, and nervous systems. [2] Psychoneuroimmunology looks at the bi-directional interplay of these systems, their involvement with emotion and behavior, and the resulting impact on health conditions including anxiety, PTSD, and autoimmunity.

Elevated levels of stress hormones suppress immunity by directly affecting cytokines. [3] Cytokines mediate the inflammatory response and contribute to neurochemical and neuroendocrine changes, which affect human physiology and behavior.

Research, while still in its infancy, shows favorable outcomes in yoga's influence on self-regulation. Yoga notably decreases mental health symptoms, while increasing tolerance and emotional awareness in comparison to highly researched psychotherapeutic and psychopharmacological interventions. [4,5,6]

Yoga has been the greatest blessing to living a life I now love.

While other modalities have also played roles in healing my life, yoga is my primary healing modality and will always be my daily spiritual practice.

We each possess our own subjective experiences, stories, and conditioning based on our individual historical life events. Yet, on an underlying level, we are all, in essence, the same.

Yoga will help you manage and heal the stress, trauma, and wounding of your past. It will remind you of who you innately are and unveil your potential capabilities. Yoga offers you a path to contribute to humanity and helps you open your heart to accept all parts of you and others.

My 3 Tips for You...

1. Keep going. It requires a concerted, repeated effort of daily practice.

2. Lean into the discomfort. The postures will reveal to you where your physical and emotional/mental pain is stored.

3. Approach your practice with curiosity and experience Yoga without judgment.

Who's Rowena?

Rowena Jayne is an adventurous, passionate woman with a love of nature, mind-body medicine, permaculture and inspirational moments. She is a Naturopath, Yoga Instructor and Trauma-informed Psychotherapist (in-training) who specializes in anxiety, trauma, emotional well-being and gut health. Rowena also authored the international best-selling book "The Joy of Real Food" which received a 5-star Indie Kurkis review, landing her on Hay House Radio, and multiple global Media Platforms.

To learn more about Rowena Jayne and all the co-authors, visit www.innerpointe.com.

References 1,2,3,4,5,6. Please see "References and Citations" in the back of the book

Cat Koo

Essay Six

"Medicine for Your Body, Mind, and Soul"

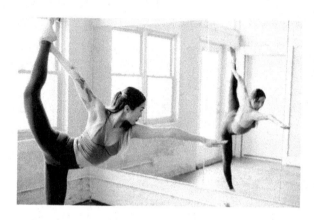

My grandfather was a doctor who worked both as a wartime medic and later as a Chinese doctor with a non-denominational temple in Hong Kong. There was no separation for me growing up between caring for the material health of a person (physical body), their emotional state, their mental state, and their spiritual and energetic body.

At the same time that I was exposed to deep spirituality, I had this very intensely material upbringing.

Such is the nature of growing up in Hong Kong. It is a place where all exists simultaneously—the hustle of global finance and trade, the roar of crickets in the humid rainforest jungle, beaches, bustling streets, and quiet mountaintops. Everything you experience and breathe exists all at the same time.

There was no conflict in understanding that all affects all. It doesn't matter if you work first on the physical body, the mental and emotional body, or your spirit. In time, it all comes together. Throughout this book, you will have read anecdotes of the profoundly transformative power of Yoga.

Physically, Yoga removes body pain and illness.

The kinds of things that we, as Yoga teachers, see in a Yoga room are the kinds of things that people describe as inspiring, healing, and miraculous; chronic back pain goes away, or knee pain dissipates. There is a student at my Yoga school who has gone from wheelchair to crutches to practicing the entire sequence of Yoga without any assistance.

Some of our students have used Yoga to heal themselves from a wide range of conditions, such as nerve pain, high blood pressure, scoliosis, arthritis, and more.

Even if going through such a dramatic physical shift is not *your story*, your personal experience is just as important and just as valid. What I do know is your physical body will just feel better from practicing Yoga.

There is, simply put, no better or more powerful health maintenance system than a regular Yoga practice in combination with a good nutritious diet. The seekers of yore and the seekers of now searched for a 'Fountain of Youth.' Here it is, as has been, for thousands of years. It is better and cheaper than any pill you can take. Moving your spine, oxygenating your blood, moving lymph, or regulating your endocrine system are only some of the most tangible things happening in Yoga.

Mahavatar Babaji taught the axiom of living life is truth, simplicity, and love. If you feel better, if something brings you joy, do more of that.

This morning, I taught Yoga to a classroom of schoolchildren, aged 6-9. Even at their age, without really knowing how or why, the young children said to me, "I feel so much more relaxed!" "I feel better!" "When will you come back and do this with us again?"

Yes! Even at that age, the children know.

Once you begin to cultivate the ability to concentrate and build an awareness of how your physical body feels, you begin to be aware of your mind. It doesn't necessarily happen in that order, but when you begin to practice being **at one**, your inner dialogue will reveal itself. Particularly, you will begin to hear the self-imposed judgments or limitations on yourself.

What are those habitual stories that you share about yourself or others and are they true, loving, and kind?

There, in the quiet of your practice, you are with your thoughts. Are you able to just be quiet and be with them? Don't beat yourself up for having "bad thoughts." Most people aren't really aware of any of it at all. Just allow yourself to be there for a moment.

Your thoughts and perceptions color your world, but they are just temporary and aren't really who you are.

When you are still enough in the present moment to feel how infinite you really are, all possibilities open up. In the present moment, even our sense of time falls away.

Healing starts in the mind. Luckily, healing is available to all. It simply begins by remembering that **you are always whole**. No one and nothing could ever take that away from you, most of all, yourself.

Healing is simply a remembrance of your truest, most expansive nature.

We, or more specifically, our pesky egos that live in our minds, can over-complicate things or step in the way. Sometimes, all Yoga does is bring your awareness to the fact that you are standing in your own way and you need not. Through the practice of Yoga, you can allow yourself to let go and begin to move at ease with the universe. When you finally allow yourself to live in harmony and joy, you will start to feel a softening of the heart.

Through awareness, you begin to be able to **notice** what affects the way you feel, think, act (or react), and live your life. The totality of how you think and feel isn't good or bad, so the first place to apply non-judgment and forgiveness is with yourself. This process of observation allows you to choose those qualities of the highest vibrations: unconditional love, forgiveness, compassion, and humility.

The actions you take are naturally affected by the quality of your thoughts and emotions.

The more you practice this, the easier it becomes. The more you allow yourself to breathe, the more you allow yourself to feel, and the more at ease you are. You begin to trust yourself enough to lead with your heart. Your natural state is a state of high health and deep connection to Spirit.

Wisdom comes from your heart, not your intellect. When you start to **become** loving kindness, you will not fret about what is the "right thing" to do in any situation because it will be clear.

Be loving awareness. Be kindness. Be your truest nature, and then you will experience great clarity in all situations, especially the most challenging ones.

Even the *attempt* at, or the thought of, being a more loving person, will impact every interaction and connection you have with every person you meet, including yourself. Love is more than a feeling or a song or a desire, hough it is all of those things too.

Love is the divine essence.

From love, comes growth, healing, and creativity. Allowing yourself to embody that essence brings you into harmony with yourself and others.

Love *instantly* shifts your consciousness away from fear, judgment, and condemnation.

From the mundane to the divine, it is the same, so it doesn't much matter what you work on first. All affects all. Whatever gifts Yoga has given you, in whatever way, whether physical, mental, emotional, or spiritual, you must practice and continue to do so without judgment of yourself. Accept where you are now, just as you would show up for anyone you love.

Your Yoga practice is a way of saying "I am here" to yourself.

Even Buddha, and all the other great masters, continued practicing meditation after attaining enlightenment. It is one thing to read something once and entirely another thing to be able to do it. One is understanding conceptually and symbolically, but the other is *knowing*.

Sometimes, being loving is too hard for people. In times of deep grief or pain, it's just such a large leap. So, start small. If being loving is just too hard, just allow yourself to feel what you do, take it all in, and at least, don't dwell on the negative.

At least, do no harm.

Gratitude is a major miracle maker. It creates a quantum shift in your being. It is the skill of seeing the world with eyes of appreciation and joy. It doesn't have to be anything big or fancy. It could be as simple as "That breath I just took was amazing!" Or being grateful for the people in your life. It makes it so much easier to see the good in yourself, and by extension, see the good in all others.

Love heals all. Love is infinite and unconditional.

See Love in all things and all people.

Peace begins *within*.

Your Yoga practice is preventative medicine for your body, mind, and soul.

Have a great class! Enjoy your practice! It's just the best.

My 3 Tips for You:

1. **The most important part of your Yoga practice is simply to practice** You must do it, even if it is not perfect, because let's face it—it will neve be.

2. **Notice what it is that you are thinking,** particularly when finishing th sentence, "I am." You are powerful, so use it for the good.

3. **Practice gratefulness.** Giving thanks offers you the opportunity t experience deep abundance and appreciation for all in life.

Who's Cat?

Cat Koo's mission is to help people create positive changes in their lives body, mind and soul in a warm and welcoming environment. She was bor and raised in Hong Kong and began practicing Yoga daily in 2005. Today Cat lives in Chicago, where she teaches Yoga and continues to practic daily at her Yoga School, Be Yoga Andersonville.

To learn more about Cat Koo and all the co-authors, visit www.innerpointe com.

Donna Rubin

Essay Seven

"Never Give Up!"

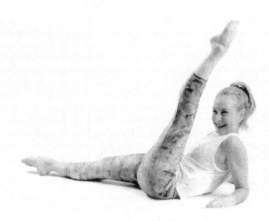

"What is Yoga?"

This is what I'd ask when I saw friends performing what appeared to be stretching exercises, but in positions that I'd never seen before. Having trained at the prestigious National Ballet School of Canada since age 12, I thought I'd seen every stretch there was.

Backstage during a performance of *Phantom of the Opera*, (I performed the principal role of Meg Giry eight times a week for four years), I noticed a fellow castmate executing odd stretches. Asking what she was doing, she responded that she was doing Yoga postures. It didn't make sense why she needed to do Yoga if she was taking ballet class every day.

Later, I witnessed this bizarre practice again when I was on the U.S. tour with the musical "Carousel." This time, my fellow castmate had the leading ballet role. Since I was desperate to eventually have the part myself, I asked her the same question. She told me she did yoga every day. Well, I figured it was about time I look into this more closely because it was now clear to me that there were benefits to this Yoga stuff that I wanted to understand.

Fast forward a year and a half to the end of the tour, and I was back in New York preparing to audition for another show. However, this time I felt different; age was catching up to me. It took longer and longer to warm up my body, and the time and effort required to prepare for auditions became less and less appealing.

It was the first time that I entertained the idea of a career transition but I was extremely concerned because I had no tangible skills other than dance!

*So, what could I possibly do at 35 years old with an increasingly uncooperative body?*I was becoming an aging dancer and lacked the formal education to pursue any other profession. Before I graduated from high school, I snagged my very first job while on holiday in NYC, a position with the San Antonio Ballet. I was so far from home but as far as I was concerned, I'd made it! Making sure that high school dropout would not be added to my resume, I quickly studied for and passed the GED.

As fate would have it, while visiting my sister in Florida, I stumbled upon Hot Yoga (Bikram Method Yoga). Without a local ballet studio, what else was there to do but finally investigate this mystery of Yoga?

I couldn't have imagined that walking into my first Yoga class would change my life.

Very quickly, I discovered that hot yoga did more to whip my body into shape than ever before. Plus, my flexibility increased, age and all! If only I had discovered this Yoga practice earlier in my career; it would have been so different.

Daily Yoga practice enabled me to control my weight, which had always been a challenge during my dance career. Classical ballet demands you look a certain way. Conforming to this 'ideal' was my biggest hurdle. Consistently, I heard from my directors that my dancing was excellent, but that I needed to lose weight, (105 pounds was still too heavy according to the powers that be). And when life events brought inevitable stress and anxiety, weight gain led to the non-renewal of my contract. There were no words to describe how much of a failure I felt.

Yoga?

Yoga, (specifically Hot Yoga), provided me with the tools to maintain my weight and break the previous habit of binging and starving. (At times, I hated my body because I could not control it).

After several months of daily Yoga classes in Florida, I realized that this new world was something very special. Not feeling judged by others, I was able to enjoy quiet time after each class, which I eventually came to understand was meditation. It meant a lot to me at the time to be part of a wonderful community that was supportive and inclusive to everyone.

The defining moment came when my sister asked, "You know Yoga so well now, why don't you teach it?"

A light bulb went off.

Teach Yoga? But I'm just a beginner!

I could do the poses, but I really knew nothing about Yoga.

Many of my colleagues pursued a career as ballet teachers, which I had considered as well, however, the competitive environment and my feeling as though I'd failed, made this option not possible.

Would teaching Yoga fulfill me as much as my performing career?Would teaching Yoga provide enough income to support me in NYC?

I figured I would give it a try.

Back in New York City, I started teaching the Yoga I'd learned in Florida to friends in a rented dance studio on Eighth Avenue. All my classes began to grow. Extremely dedicated, I practiced and taught every day. In time, I became certified as a Bikram Yoga instructor. At teacher training, I spent nine weeks immersed in daily Yoga, listening to these mantras…

« Never underestimate yourself."

« Don't let anyone steal your peace."

Through practice, I was able to still my mind, listen to my true self, and begin to see life differently. The message was getting louder and clearer every day.

Yoga not only gives you a great workout and helps you become more flexible; it's also about learning to calm and guide your mind, opening the door to your truest desires, and to the realization that you are okay, just the way you are.

There came a turning point when I realized that there was more to yoga practice than was first obvious…

After each floor posture, my teacher would say, "Turn around, lie down, and don't move." I was listening carefully and doing what I was told to do. However, one day, I realized that every time I was in Savasana, I moved around and stretched more. I didn't even realize that I was doing this and thought the words did not apply to me. At the time, I thought doing more was being a better yogi.

The day I realized that I was not listening was the day I understood why I was being asked to remain still.

Being, rather than *doing,* was ultimately where the real benefits of yoga lay. **Wow!**

The simple realization of how difficult it was to stay still, and how difficult it was to just *be* instead of *do*, was mind-blowing.

I get it! I get it! Yes!

That's why I feel so good after yoga class.

I am okay just the way I am.

Nowhere to go, nothing to do, just BE.

It was through the benefits of yoga that I truly believe I was able to make seamless transitions—from a performer to a yoga teacher, to the owner of multiple yoga studios.

Why wasn't there an official Hot Yoga Studio in New York City? It was absurd! There were a handful of studios in the United States at that time, but not in New York City! Certainly, Broadway and ballet dancers would benefit from it.

Even though I knew nothing about business and was a relatively new teacher on the New York Yoga scene, my practice gave me the direction, strength, and courage to go for it. As fate had it, I was even able to convince a landlord to give me a lease—with no business plan and no business history.

Lucky to find someone that shared my belief in Yoga, the stars were aligned, and the perfect business partner appeared to help open the first studio in the theater district. In just eight months, it was so successful that I was able to repay my investor all of the start-up funds. Due to a growing demand or Yoga, she then joined me full-time to help expand by adding additional studios. We were able to provide classes every hour to accommodate every student's schedule. This model had never been done before, and I figured if it worked for me, it would work for everyone. After all, New York is the city that never sleeps!

Now, after 24 years, and at one time seven studios, I've come to a point where my once primary passion to own and operate Yoga studios has shifted. Unlike the majority of other Yoga practices, Hot Yoga was the best place for me to start because, in this seemingly 'non-Yoga' class, I was able to practice without being required to chant words I did not understand and sit in the lotus position to meditate. In other words, as a former dancer, I understood a focus on the physical, but spiritual practice was another matter.

It was this simple beginner's class that started my journey within, and now I am in transition again.

I've found a new passion. The Covid-19 pandemic gave me the extra time to listen anew to my inner voice, to be open to fresh ways of thinking and teaching that give emotional and psychic space to those who have suffered trauma, and how to reach them in a fully compassionate way. Now diving into studying Mindfulness-Based-Stress-Reduction, I'm discovering whole new insights and ideas for myself and those I work with.

If you get anything from this essay, perhaps discover that transitions in life are normal and navigable. With yoga, mindfulness, and the right nudges along the way, you can go *within* and gracefully move through the next steps in your life.

My 3 Tips for You...

1. Listen to your inner voice.

2. Approach your life and practice with compassion.

3. NEVER GIVE UP!

Who's Donna?

Donna Rubin is a life-long performer who's dedicated to supporting others in the arts. As a former professional dancer, she performed with the National Ballet of Canada, principal role of "Meg Giry" in the original Canadian company of Phantom of the Opera, and later made her Broadway debut in Carousel at Lincoln Center. In 1999, Donna cofounded multi-location bodē NYC, New York's first hot yoga studio.

To learn more about Donna Rubin and all the co-authors, visit www.innerpointe.com.

Nadine Faitas

Essay Eight

"The Gripping Tale of Self-Discovery and Never Giving Up"

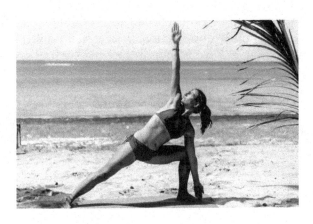

For so long, I was content and happy with my life, or so I thought. The greatest fear was losing everything that mattered to me, especially my husband, who was my world. Freshly married and madly in love after a five-year long-distance relationship between Germany and Italy, we finally lived together in Munich. Losing him would be the end of me, or so I believed.

Then, one summer day, my nightmare became a reality. My husband went missing, and my family and the police searched for him everywhere.

I knew something terrible must have happened.

Until I got a phone call from my best friend: "Nadine," she said, "you must be very strong now. The police found your husband, and he is not injured but lost his memory and has no idea who he is." At that very moment, I felt like dying. The pain and helplessness I felt were unbearable. What did she mean? He lost his memory and didn't know who he was.

On my way back from a business trip, I was about to board a plane from Hamburg to Munich. I don't remember much of the flight or the time between the phone call and arriving at the hospital. It felt like I was standing beside myself, watching me, but still fully being there. The nurse guided me into the emergency room, where he lay in a bed. I walked slowly toward him, and the moment his eyes caught mine, I knew he didn't know who I was.

The eyes that looked at me full of love for all these years were empty, lonely, sad, and confused.

Five years passed, during which I tried to help him back into life. He slowly regained his memory from zero to the day they found him, to remembering probably all the facts he has ever learned in school or life. Over time, he also remembered his family and friends. But he had no recollection of our love story, how we met, our wedding, or the time we had spent together. I was a stranger to him.

Time passed, and it became normal to wake up to someone who looked like my husband and behaved like him but wasn't him anymore. Over the years, I became a mixture of a housemate, friend, and mother but not a wife. Losing him was always my biggest fear. But the worst thing ever that happened to me was that I lost myself.

Over these years, I focused entirely on him, helping him get his life and career back, supporting and waiting for him to remember me. But I lost myself in the process. It probably started three years after his amnesia. Incredible sadness sunk in, and I didn't know where it came from. Hardly able to hold myself together at work, I found myself crying every night, unable to stop.

I blamed my husband and wished he could help me. I kept hoping he would find a way to love me again, like before. But he was lost too, and I had to accept that.

Getting promoted in my corporate job didn't help the situation. The pressure and the new responsibility added anxiety to my sadness. Feeling lost, stressed, and sad, I didn't know what to do. This is when my real Yoga journey started! One day, I couldn't live this life anymore. I was no longer able to do this job that I hated all day, return home to my husband, fight with him in the evening, and cry myself to sleep.

Eventually, in 2017, I took a sabbatical and attended the Bikram Yoga Teacher Training in Acapulco. The experience was life-changing, and I felt better than I had in years. I didn't cry once in the three months of the training, except for the day of graduation, when...

...I realized my time in the Yoga bubble was over, and I had to face reality

gain.

When I returned from training, I got a job offer in London. It seemed like that was the perfect solution to my problems. So, I accepted, and three months later moved to the UK. My intention was not to leave my husband but to get some space. But this wasn't the solution either. Leaving Munich, my husband, and my family to escape the pressures of my old life only led to a personal breakdown and finally ended our relationship.

After months of not knowing what was wrong with me, being sad, and experiencing sleep deprivation, I got diagnosed with depressive anxiety disorder. There was no moment of happiness or joy—not even when my beautiful nephew was born. As I began grieving the loss of my husband and the future that I had envisioned for us, my healing journey started. After spending six months of hell in London, alone in a big city without my family or friends during the biggest crisis of my life, and having suicidal thoughts every day on my way to work…

…I made a decision. The decision that I wanted to be happy!

This decision changed everything. Beginning a daily Yoga practice helped me to start smiling again. Delving into personal development, spirituality, and mindset books, I attended live seminars led by Tony Robbins. My internal turmoil began to dissipate even more when I walked on hot coals. Traveling to India, I spent time in an Ashram without speaking for days. I learned how to go *within,* meditate, and be still with my thoughts.

All of these things helped me to understand myself better.

I discovered my thoughts weren't facts and were causing my sadness. It was liberating to realize I didn't have to believe them all.

Practicing in the hot room helped to deepen that new understanding. After practicing Bikram Yoga for over ten years, I finally understood its true essence. Yoga became my 90-minute open-eye meditation. You face yourself in the mirror, your true self, with all your dark sides, and whatever thoughts that come up, you don't have to listen. Focus on your breath. Focus on the teacher's voice guiding you. Focus on your body and the postures. If your mind tells you it's too hot and you must leave the room, ask your body if that's true.

You will notice you have your tools.

One tool is your breath. Once you focus on that, your heartbeat will slow down. (This works, by the way, for anxiety or stress). Whenever you feel stressed or nervous, focus on your breath and slow it down. Breathe out longer than you inhale. You will see it works magic.

It's all about having tools! They exist, and you must find the right ones for you. My biggest lesson is that you can heal any trauma once you find your tools! For myself, the most extensive trauma was when my husband lost his memory.

But losing myself almost cost me my life.

A year after I decided to be happy, I quit my cooperate job, divorced, and sold everything I had. I started traveling the world. During my travels, I got to teach my favorite Bikram Yoga in over 30 studios in 20 different countries. During the past three years, I got to know myself better and better by practicing Bikram Yoga, Vipassana, and Breathwork. I tried different therapies and healing methods, such as family constellations, sound healings, kundalini activation sessions, cacao ceremonies, and ecstatic dance. Several coaches, from mindset to spiritual to business coaches, helped me better understand myself and become the best version of myself.

Almost everything on my bucket list came true. While traveling to over 30 countries, I swam with dolphins and learned how to surf. During my year in Kenya, I went on safaris, where I saw the big five and climbed the top of Mount Kenya. Starting to reconnect with my femininity, I began to dance ballet again. In Peru, I experienced that our essence is pure love during an Ayahuasca ceremony. Eventually, I found a new home in Portugal, where I live now. An incredible place by the beach, more beautiful than I could ever dream of during my depression in rainy London.

In hindsight, I realized what caused the sadness for all those years in my "old life" and cooperate career was that I had no purpose. To help others transform their lives as I did, I became a certified strategic intervention life coach. As a Bikram Yoga Teacher and Coach, I help others become the happiest and best versions of themselves by helping them understand their bodies and minds.

My breakup was a wake-up call to go within and find myself.

Sometimes a breakup can feel like the end of the world, but it's just the beginning of a new chapter in your life. Use this opportunity to find yourself, heal your wounds, and discover the path that leads to your best life.

My journey of self-discovery taught me that the only person I could make appy was myself. It was a hard lesson, but I'm glad I learned it. I no longer ely on external factors to bring me joy, and I'm grateful for every moment. found myself again, and in doing so, I found a happiness that I never hought was possible.

The human spirit is powerful.

Going *within* helps us discover the true essence of who we are. Often to ind answers, it›s almost a rite of passage that we must first experience deep painful moments in life. And perhaps it is the pain that is opening us o self-discovery and the power to never give up.

My 3 Tips for You...

1. When you think you have been buried, you might just have been planted.

2. Be curious to explore yourself and your emotions; allow yourself to feel all the emotions; that's why you are here.

3. Remember, what doesn't kill you makes you stronger.

Who's Nadine?

Nadine Faitas combines Strategic Intervention Coaching with Yoga and Mindfulness to help people better understand themselves. She discovered Bikram Yoga in Hamburg in 2007, struck by its transformative power. Shortly after she started practicing, during a sabbatical, she became a certified instructor. She realized it's not just about us, but also about serving a greater purpose.

To learn more about Nadine Faitas and all the co-authors, visit www.innerpointe.com.

Adrianne "Ajax" Jackson

Essay Nine

"Empowerment Through Yoga"

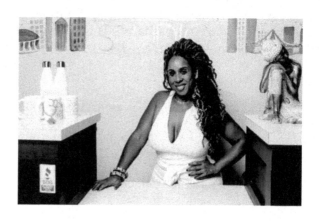

Early on, I learned that a Yoga practice is one of the most intimate things a person can have, like the lace underwear in your underwear drawer.

It's delicate, personal, stretched, and tailored just for you.

This essay is focused on one sweet side to Yoga, and that's the empowerment side anyone can discover in their own practice. An empowered life is one of the most precious gifts you can receive from Yoga and where I personally teach and live from.

My parents are geniuses.

Born in Los Angeles, California at Cedars Sinai in Beverly Hills, I identify as a Black Latina woman, specifically Mexican and Black. My mother is Mexican, and my father was Black. Both hardworking, smart, and loving, they raised my sister and me with an incredible upbringing that included the best in education, neighborhoods, classes, healthcare, travel, language, community, art, and culture.

What they were able to provide and expose to me and my sister was divinely orchestrated by their hard work, planning, and desiring the best for their daughters. We are so grateful. These riches from our parents included the remarkable healing art of Yoga.

Through hard work and education, my parents advanced in their lives. As avid readers, they had an extensive book collection that I grew up looking through. There were subjects we never discussed at home, but I learned about them by reading their books. It seemed as if our parents were divinely inspired because there was one of my father's books that kept drawing my attention for years.

I stared at the front and back cover year after year, but I felt I was never ready to open this particular book. At the same time, every time I picked up the book, I would experience this strange unexplainable sense of clarity that one day, I would be ready to open it. The funny thing is, although I never opened the Yoga book, I did open the *Joy of Sex* and the *Joy of Cooking*!

This book, "Autobiography of a Yogi" by Paramahansa Yogananda, would eventually turn out to be life-changing for me.

Later, I discovered that this book influenced countless people, including Steve Jobs and Kareem Abdul Jabbar. Both of them considered Paramahansa Yogananda's words to be transformative in their lives. At Steve Jobs's funeral service, a copy of the book was given to everyone in attendance. Kareem has said that Yoga kept him injury-free for years in the NBA. Countless people have been deeply transformed by this book.

Eventually, "Autobiography of a Yogi" came back into my life in a most auspicious way. It was there when I went to Yoga teacher training in 2008. Of course, I read the book from cover to cover during nine weeks of intensive training.

The time and place in this book felt familiar, from either my dreams or perhaps even a past life.

Eventually ending up in Kolkata, India in 2015, I retraced some of Paramahansa's footsteps that he wrote about, including ending up at the Ghosh family home where Mukunda Ghosh (Paramahansa) was raised. With a sense of wonder and awe, this put me in the meditation room where he found God.

Wanting to deepen my own practice and teaching skills, I took a special training at the Ghosh Yoga College of India. It was led directly by Paramahansa's great-niece, Muktamala Mitra. She is a fierce, sassy, striking, and remarkable woman and Yogi. Oftentimes, she would find me hiding away at school, studying and practicing Yoga. Being in India was powerful, mystical, and challenging, and helped me connect to the legacy and Yoga experience that continues to influence me today.

All of my Yoga trainings empowered me and changed the trajectory of my life.

After several years of teaching and practicing Yoga, the mission I was on became more deeply defined. In 2016, through a culmination of almost a decade of work, Magnolia Yoga Studio was created; the first Black-owned Yoga studio in Louisiana! Our business model is focused on diversity, inclusivity, and affordability in Yoga. This created a brand-new clientele base of mostly African American women, many doing Yoga for the first time. Our clientele and fan base grows, and people of all backgrounds are attracted to the studio near the French Quarter in New Orleans. Essentially, people who are in the shadows—unspoken of, unspoken to, and in a way, left to fend for themselves in the world, are showing up to begin their journey into Yoga.

It has become vital to remove the barriers to accessing wellness solutions like Yoga, regardless of race, size, orientation, or economic status. Remarkable shifts happen when we prioritize our *most* vulnerable groups.

Other vulnerable and underrepresented people feel curious and comfortable to come and be amongst the loving, healing vibes and environment found in Yoga. Having a safe place to practice helps to heal from trauma and despair, gently guiding us to a loving experience *within*.

The power of these tools is available to anyone who seeks them.

Keep in mind, Yoga is a way of life; it is a practice and it has its own process for each person.

For many, Yoga improves their sleep, which can lead to significant improvements in mood, repair, and focus. For others, their breathing capacity and awareness double. Some students report their mobility and circulation improve and navigating the world seems less daunting, restrictive, and exhausting.

Small, yet significant, changes add up for people. They become compelled to do something with their newfound energy, insights, mood, and mobility, which is how Yoga can help us all lead a very fulfilling life.

Yoga practice is an experience that starts on the mat but gets played out in everyday life with big and small decisions, actions, words, and behaviors. Some students often receive what appears to be instant healing for both physical and emotional challenges.

Yoga is therapy; it is a medicine, an alternative to pain, pills, depression, and suffering. It helps us remove and heal physical, mental, and emotional barriers and blocks, which allows for balance, prevention, union, increased life force, reduced stress, more consciousness, and sustainability.

Technically, the teacher is only there to guide students through the process of acquiring these benefits. In other words, a teacher helps the student see what is true for them. Essentially, a student realizes how their life is unfolding and what is right for them. These are some of the internal truths and dynamics experienced in Yoga, a word that comes from the Sanskrit language meaning "union."

Yoga empowerment can spark creativity and place your destiny into your hands through optimal health and wellness.

Self-awareness, another side effect of Yoga, is an ability to understand self, and the various aspects of who you are; from how your mind works, to your body, your emotions, and your energy. Self-awareness can be gained in many ways. A Yoga practice for many has been the most direct and less painful method to self-awareness.

The personal development rate for self-awareness varies for each person. It's always best to focus *within*, on your own insights, rather than comparing yourself with someone else. However, the more self-awareness you build and practice, the more you can elevate your experiences in life.

When your heart and mind are open, people will want to work with you, be around you, and ultimately, be inspired to build their own levels of self-awareness.

One of my favorite things about Yoga and why I am always confident in recommending it to people is its direct nature. In a world still filled with discrimination, oppression, and politics, Yoga does not pick favorites and does not skip you in line or overlook you. If you do Yoga, you will receive the benefits, no matter who you are and at whatever level you start.

Perhaps these insights will inspire you to jump onto a Yoga mat and explore what is possible for you!

My 3 Tips for You...

1. Travel far and more often. Yoga is an inner journey, and at some point, taking your Yoga skills out into the world is very important! So, travel— the further, the better!

2. A good Yoga practice is a consistent Yoga practice. Meaning, you don't have to be good at Yoga, just be consistent at doing it; from there, the magic

will follow.

3. Lean into the uncomfortable, whether it's conversations, people experiences, work, classes, or places—that is where your next level *within* wants to develop.

Who's Ajax?

Adrianne "Ajax" Jackson is owner of Magnolia Yoga Studio, the first Black-owned Yoga Studio in Louisiana. She is multi-lingual visionary community change maker and a wellness programming pioneer. Ajax was awarded the 2020 Visionary Award for her commitment to diversity. She believes passionately in the human potential and her commitment to people's wellness is what motivates her every day.

To learn more about Adrianna "Ajax" Jackson and all the co-authors, visit www.innerpointe.com.

John Salvatore

Essay Ten

"Treat Yourself with Love"

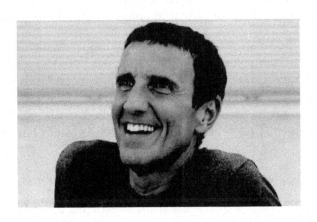

At sixteen years old, I became a professional performer and started an incredible career onstage. Work would—and often still does—involve appearing onstage eight times a week, with only one day off to rest.

To perform at this level, the body needs to be maintained, which initially involved working out at the gym, often with such discipline that I would find my routine consisted of workout to stage, day after day.

That was my routine.

I would always be on the go, which in those early days would mean dancing and performing, working out at the gym, a new fitness class to get into—and coexisting with this, drinking, partying, and other distractions. I was living life at 150% and constantly pushing myself.

During this period, friends would suggest that I try Yoga and for years I resisted. I just didn't think it would be my thing. Until one day in 1999, while on the stair-master at the gym, a friend told me that if I would give it a shot, I would really love it. She pointed out a yoga studio that was right up the street, (this was mid-town in NYC) where they heated the room to 105°F and you sweat!

"The best workout you'll ever have!"

As soon as the words, "best workout you'll ever have!" and "sweat!" passed her lips, I jumped off the stair master, ran from the gym, and headed straight to the Yoga studio.

My first teacher was Donna Rubin, who, as it turned out, had also been a dancer—a ballet dancer. Could this be what I was looking for?

I was never very good at meditating because it was tough for me to sit still. But I came to realize that Yoga would come to ultimately calm my mind.

In 1993, I became sober after years of struggling with alcohol and cocaine addiction. The chosen method of quieting the "voices in my head" had now been removed. But for 90 minutes, in the Yoga studio, those voices would become quiet, leaving me simply with my breath and a new-found peace. The thoughts that had previously filled my head, were gone. I learned later that while practicing, our nervous system balances out, and the mind calms.

I began to understand that Yoga could help those in sobriety.

Yoga had me hooked, and I went from practicing three times a week to virtually every day. Yoga was not only contributing to my sobriety but also helped me as a dancer, physically and mentally. Donna suggested that I might try the teacher training course; there weren't very many male teachers at the time. I hadn't considered teaching up to that point, yet after some consideration, I saw that perhaps this might be exactly what I wanted to do and in 2001, I was blessed to receive a $5,000 "Career Transition for Dancers" grant from the Actors Equity Union to help pay for the course.

Practicing Yoga is a gift to yourself. It gets you out of your own way...

...by exposing emotional memories which are accessed and then released through many Yoga postures, moving through vulnerability, to an opening of the chakras, and finally to a sense of peace and serenity. Through this sometimes-uncomfortable journey, we learn to use our breath. We breathe.

Sometimes it might even feel like pain because the mind doesn't always know the difference between discomfort and deeper physical pain. When practicing Yoga (or really anytime in life) it's important to always treat your body and mind with love and respect. Only do what you can at any given time. Avoid causing unnecessary trauma to yourself. Learning to breathe through the mental, emotional, and physical sensations will allow the mind to remain calm, so you can be aware of what is actually happening.

A little slice of my own journey...

Since the age of five, I knew that I was gay. Back in the 1960s, that was a subject that was never discussed. Much of my childhood was lost because I was trying to be the person that everybody else thought I would/should be, instead of the person I knew I was. My father was a conservative lawyer, and having a gay son was often very difficult for him.

By eighth grade, I realized that I wanted to be an actor and a dancer. One of my English teachers had been a performer on Broadway for years and became a mentor, guiding me toward my dream of performing.

He made me believe that I could be anyone I wanted to be, without fear.

Taking the plunge, I started to get parts in school plays and soon after, to get jobs in summer stock. I found myself immersed in dance and acting classes. My dad was unaware of this, but every week, my mom would give up some of her grocery money to pay for my classes. Her encouragement helped me to understand that I was okay and that the world could be a safe place after all.

A Father's Love

Over the years, I've been blessed to have had many roles in many productions. For eight years, I performed in *Jersey Boys* in Las Vegas. During this run, Bob Durkin, the first director/choreographer to hire me as a kid, came to see me in the show. Afterward, we talked for a while and he shared with me something that my late father had told him.

Bob explained that Dad was worried about letting me go into show business; that I may not have what it takes to enter such a ruthless profession in which not many people could make a living. Bob replied, *"You have to let him go because he has what it takes."*

Injuries and Letting Go

Over the years, due to my "occupational hazard" as a dedicated dancer, I have gone through many injuries and consequently, many surgeries. In 2006, while on tour with *Hairspray*, I had to take a leave of absence due to arthritis in my hips. For a period of time, I would go back and forth from the show to hot yoga to help me keep performing. More doctors, then more yoga.

Eventually, I discovered that I was learning the same lesson over and over until I could get it right. In my mind, I was still trying to act like I was moving and dancing like I was in my teens and 20s. I was essentially competing with myself. Learning how to grow gracefully and letting go of what is no longer meant for me, is who I am today.

My new mantra is this… be kind to your body, respect your body, take care of your body, and most of all, *learn to let go.*

The heat in Yoga becomes your best friend

The yoga room is hot. You'll always deal with the heat—everybody's dealing with the heat. And the heat becomes your best friend. You can fight it, or you can surrender and embrace whatever comes your way in a hot Yoga room.

Each day, Yoga is a new beginning. Every time that you come out of class, there's that feeling and sense of self-confidence. By going *within,* self-awareness and a new perspective reveal themselves to you each time.

Yoga helps you to deal with any situation that can come up in life. Equanimity in the face of adversity.

I'll finish as I started….

"Treat Yourself with Love"

My 3 Tips for You…

1. Treat yourself with love and compassion.

2. Always breathe calmly, with awareness.

3. Use the mirrors in your life as a reflection of love.

Who's John?

John Salvatore started Yoga in 1999. After practicing for 18 months, he knew that Yoga was going to be part of his life forever. Performing on stage for years as an actor and dancer on Broadway and in Las Vegas, he took a short sabbatical to become certified in Bikram Yoga in 2001. Today, John continues to teach in NYC and in other studios in the U.S and around the world.

To learn more about John Salvatore and all the co-authors, visit www.innerpointe.com.

Deborah Small

Essay Eleven

"When You're Willing to Change Your Point of View, the Things You Look at Change."

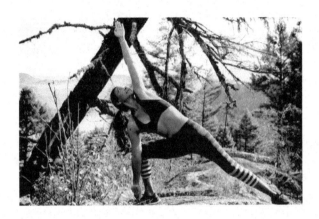

This chapter looks at how adopting a Yoga and Meditation discipline can help you change your point of view, using the body and the breath as a medium. In this chapter, I will share what it did for me and what it can do for you in your daily life, beyond the physical benefits.

The physical aspects of yoga are like a bridge that creates awareness of subconscious patterns. This allows you to become conscious of the patterns you have stored within you; the behavioral patterns that drive your choices.

Yoga provides you with the tools needed to enable your Self to change subconsciously-held viewpoints; revealing positive changes in the perceived world. It can open up a whole new vista of life for you; all as a consequence of practicing yoga.

ABOUT ME: I was born in Cape Town, South Africa, and raised in a township comprising colored people during the Apartheid era. I was the oldest of seven children. My father was a fisherman, and my mother was a homemaker.

I believe I experienced a very normal childhood and was loved and protected by my parents and extended family and community.

SPIRITUALITY: My earliest recollection of spirituality was through my Christian upbringing where I was introduced to the concept of 'God.' From an early age, I was very curious about God; that curiosity was essentially my first connection to spirituality.

Today, for me, **spirituality is the ability to connect with the God consciousness *within* myself** and to see God in all.

AWARENESS: One of my earliest memories is from when I was around three years old. My mother was getting me dressed one morning; she was putting my favorite dress on me and struggled to get the dress over my head. After she got the dress on, I lifted my head up and said to her, "I think this dress is shrinking," but my mother answered, "No, you are growing."

Just like that, at that moment, my Self became aware that I had a body. I experienced real awareness for the first time.

FEAR: My first recollection of feeling fear was my first day at school. It was the first time I was away from family and in a classroom setting with strangers. The teacher handed us crayons and paper and instructed us to draw a picture. I don't recall ever drawing before that and felt afraid that I wouldn't be able to do it. I attempted to draw a house with trees and my family, but after looking at all the other children's pictures in comparison, I decided that my picture was not as good as theirs and I was clearly not good at drawing. Creating and harboring this belief acted as a kind of protective mechanism for me at the time, but the result was that I struggled throughout most of my school life.

MISTAKE: My self-esteem/self-worth became affected by my interpretation of that event and others like it. I had created a subconscious belief by associating self-worth with achievement.

This is an example of how we subconsciously create beliefs and find evidence to support them. We create subconscious programs and patterns quite innocently and they become our 'truths' for the rest of our lives, unless or until we bring awareness to them.

Through cultivating a daily yoga and meditation practice, I was able to recognize that my self-worth isn't related to what I do, but that **I am worthy just because I am**.

CONSCIOUS/SUBCONSCIOUS: 95% of life is run from the subconscious and only 5% from our conscious mind [*cite: Dr. Bruce Lipton*].

Over time, I discovered that most of my life was lived by my subconscious patterns. My yoga and meditation practice created stillness and allowed for my stories, attachments, fears, and "coping mechanisms" to be exposed.

I'm grateful to my younger Self for creating coping mechanisms to help me survive. I had done the best I could with the mechanisms I had, but I now no longer needed some of them.

Subconscious programming starts *in utero* and is fully formed by the time we are 6-7 years old. All of it is learned unconsciously from our environment and stored in the subconscious mind.

There's a good reason for this; it's called efficiency. Our brains utilize the path of least resistance and the most energy-efficient way to function. The subconscious mind can process up to 20 million bits of information per second, and the conscious mind only has 40 bits of information per second [cite: Dr. Bruce Lipton].

Basic programming functionality need not be relearned, like walking and talking. These are the positive subconscious programs.

What we do want to become aware of are the patterns, habits, and coping mechanisms that we developed that no longer serve us or now cause pain and suffering.

MINDFUL — BE PRESENT: Eventually, I understood that my subconscious programmed thoughts were running my life.

In order to live a positive, better life, I became committed to changing those thought patterns. Whenever my mind wanted to create a negative story, I found something positive to replace it with. **By becoming mindful and being present, I was more successful in bringing about the needed change.**

The more I practiced it, the easier it became. Just like a muscle, you have to exercise it over and over to strengthen it.

PAIN & SUFFERING: Pain and suffering can work as a tool or catalyst to create change.

For example, in my early 20s, I was a single mother struggling emotionally, financially, and physically. The responsibility weighed heavily. I grieved for the life I had dreamt of having, thus creating a lot of pain and suffering for myself.

Experiencing that drove me to seek help, and as they say, "When the student is ready, the teacher will appear." A friend told me about a breathing class that had many scientific health benefits. She didn't mention meditation or yoga, just that I could learn some breathing techniques that would teach me how to access more of my lung capacity and increase my energy levels. Who doesn't want more energy?

That weeklong course became the catalyst for changing the entire trajectory of my life. I was introduced to yoga and meditation, which turned into a lifelong journey toward self-realization.

HEALING: After experiencing that course, I started a daily meditation practice. I also became more interested in exploring yoga and all of its benefits. Soon thereafter, I decided to attend yoga teacher training. I wanted to make the world a better place by sharing all the benefits. There is a saying, "If you want to learn more about something, teach it."

HOT YOGA: When I moved to North America a few years later, I was introduced to Bikram Yoga by a friend. After living my life in warmer climates, I was struggling to adjust to the cold winters in British Columbia, Canada, where we settled. My friend thought this hot yoga class would help me adjust to the cold weather better.

During my first class, I thought I was going to die! It's very normal to feel overwhelmed during your first class because of the heat and humidity conditions and the 90 minutes duration it takes to complete the sequence of 26 postures and two breathing exercises. Although the first class was tough, I remained curious and came back for a second class.

I have been practicing consistently for the past 17 years, as a student and later as a teacher.

When I think back on what made me fall in love with this practice, I can say it's the deep connection I felt to myself during the Savasana (also known as corpse pose) posture at the end of the class. You become quite still because of the exhaustion, and in this stillness comes the opportunity to connect to your true Self.

The busy mind is finally quiet; there are no distractions, allowing you to become aware of the present moment. The only thing that's left is YOU.

ARRIVAL: I can truly say that practicing and teaching yoga, combined with a daily meditation routine, has helped me to live my life with more ease, joy, and glory. Every day holds a new opportunity to take another step forward on the journey toward myself.

When you take total responsibility for your life you can become totally free to create the life you are worthy of; all it needs is a commitment to yourself. When you do this, everyone around you will benefit.

YOU: If you're reading this and you feel like your life is a struggle, make a commitment to yourself today and start a yoga and meditation practice. You've got nothing to lose and everything to gain.

My 3 Tips for You...

1. Don't delay; start where you are today.

2. Don't make the mistake to compare yourself to others.

3. The day you start, you will improve physically, mentally, and emotionally.

Who's Deborah?

Deborah Small is an internationally acknowledged practitioner of holistic healing with more than two decades of global practical experience. She holds several qualifications, including Bikram Yoga Teacher, Family Constellation Facilitator, Nutritionist and Advanced Breathing and Meditation Instructor. Deborah is a renowned motivational speaker, retreat facilitator and holds a degree in psychology from University of British Columbia.

To learn more about Deborah Small and all the co-authors, visit www.innerpointe.com.

Anurag Choudhury

Essay Twelve

"Endless Possibilities"

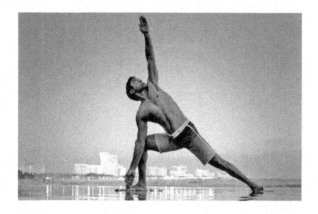

Growing up in a global yoga family, I did not always like to practice yoga.

To be completely honest, I thought it was boring. I always appreciated the workout aspect of it but never understood how it could help and provide benefits in life. As I grew older, this significantly changed. If I was really stressed out, or having a bad day, I would go take a Bikram Yoga class and instantly feel better.

Why was this?

After Yoga, I was always reminded to slow down and take life one day at a time. Life can definitely be short, but it can also be very long, just like in class. Some Yoga classes feel like an eternity, and other classes feel like a breeze. One asana at a time, there's no need to rush. The length of the class does not change, but how busy your mind is will determine how long the class takes. This has helped me learn how to not overthink situations. There's not much you can control in life besides your decisions and actions. Good and bad things will always occur. Not knowing when they will happen is what makes life interesting.

Being the son of two renowned yoga teachers, you feel obligated to continue in your parents' footsteps. But what I have learned is that obligation is not enough. I needed to discover my purpose on my own. It is a never-ending journey we all face.

The pursuit of purpose. *Yoga has acted as a guide and a blueprint for how to live my life.*

Yoga has been so much more than a physical practice. It's been a way of life that I was born into. As a child, I grew up in a Yoga studio. I spent more time there than most children would probably like to. When you're a kid, you try to have fun out of nothing. Some of my best memories were setting up skate ramps with tables and launching myself into the pile of hundreds of extra towels the studio kept in the back storage rooms. I didn't see it then, but today I see it more as a blessing than a burden.

As I grew older, I started to appreciate Yoga so much more. When you are born into Yoga, you don't get to find it on your own.

Find what?

As an adult, when you start your Yoga journey and discover the benefits it comes with, it usually hits you immediately. This is something I had to experience on my own. I was 14 years old when I tore cartilage in my knee. I went to multiple doctors and quickly had surgery scheduled. I was heavily into sports and needed to recover quickly. When I finally told my father about the scheduled surgery, he told me to cancel it and get my ass into the hot room. I listened to him and that was the first time in my life I began to consistently practice Bikram Yoga.

To this day, I've never had any more knee problems.

Yoga has been around for so long that people interpret it in different ways. If you ask me, there is nothing wrong with that. It actually makes it more special. Yoga can be whatever you want it to be. It can be anything, or it can be nothing, but it is everything.

You're doing yoga every second of your life. When you move, breathe, think, talk, and sleep, you're doing a form of Yoga.

In today's world, we have grown to believe Yoga is one thing, or one way, which is stretching—commonly known as Hatha Yoga—but it is so much more. It is widely known as a physical practice, but it can also be mental, spiritual, and emotional to name a few. It can even be evil, if you really think about it.

How is this possible?

Because if you're not careful, it can lead you on a path of destruction. Yoga can also lead you on a path of bliss. That's the beauty of it. By going *within* you get to choose.

You get to decide what you want Yoga to be.

My main focus as a Yoga teacher has always been to introduce people to what Yoga can be other than a physical practice. Growing up in the United States, many people have no idea what Yoga is. Even my closest friends do not know what Yoga is other than stretching. While this is definitely true and a big part of an individual's Yoga practice, there is so much more to learn.

You are doing Yoga every second of your existence.

This is something I learned from my parents and intend to share with the world. I believe once people begin to see this side of Yoga, they will open unimaginable doors.

Throughout my life, my personal Yoga practice has been sporadic. I have learned that this is normal. Things are always going to change. As long as you do not give up, and eventually find the time, you will be rewarded. The same goes for my Yoga teaching career. I started to teach Bikram Yoga at the age of 23. As a young Yoga teacher, I did not teach as much as I could, having had many other interests and goals I wanted to achieve. However, after I taught my first few classes, I decided I was going to teach Yoga for the rest of my life. I plan on teaching much more consistently as I get older.

Yoga can help you with so many things in life.

Yoga can help you daily with stress, concentration, and problem-solving. As humans, we are fighting with distractions every day. Distractions can directly affect the outcome of any situation. This is why I believe learning how to concentrate and focus on the task at hand is one of the most important tools to learn in life. It can make or break you in any situation. This is something we all have an equal chance to learn.

Growing up in a Yoga studio, I was able to witness so many people transform their physical, emotional, and mental well-being through the practice of Yoga. This has been one of the biggest blessings in my life. Witnessing this firsthand ultimately encouraged me to continue in my parents' footsteps as a Yoga teacher.

I truly believe a Yoga practice can help motivate you to live a healthier and improved life. By showing up to class, you create a sense of discipline and focus that can help in all aspects of life.

And the best part?

You lose nothing by trying. Even if it's not for you, simply showing up is a valuable step in the right direction.

Showing up to class is the most important part of it all. The possibilities are endless and the doors that open are infinite with the practice of Yoga.

My 3 Tips for You...

1. *Breathing.* Understanding your breath is a never-ending process. Your breath controls everything. Learning to listen to it, follow it, and control it can significantly change your Yoga practice. If you learn to control your breath, you can control your life.

2. *Patience.* Every class is different; some are going to be good and some are going to be bad. Don't get discouraged because your body is not allowing itself to do things you were doing in a previous class. Yoga is a long-term investment.

3. *Trying the right way.* Yoga is not always about perfecting the posture, but trying the right way will lead to benefits. Even if you cannot do certain postures to perfection, the journey of trying to do it the right way will maximize your practice.

Who's Anurag?

Growing up in a yoga-centered household, Anurag was inspired to become a yoga teacher. He has a passion for producing music, TV, and film, and enjoys exploring real estate and finance. Additionally, Anurag enjoys creative pursuits like writing and photography, making him a multifaceted individual.

To learn more about Anurag and all the co-authors, visit www.innerpointe.com.

Mica Fish

Essay Thirteen

"The Art of Manifesting
The Life You Want to Live"

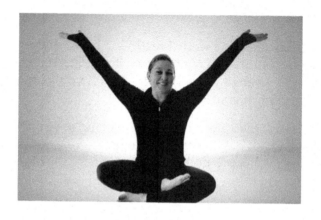

From Breaking My Ankles to Building an Empire: How My Yoga Practice is the Catalyst for Creating the Life of My Dreams

But, let's rewind; it wasn't always this way.

Being in terrible condition, I first found a Hot 26 & 2 Yoga class as a young 20-something. Physically, I was in a lot of pain. I was injured from a passionate snowboarding career and had a terrible self-destructive relationship with my body.

Emotionally, I was a wreck. I was stuck on a merry-go-round of ingesting the trending antianxiety medications and suffering daily all the flat affect and roller coaster side effects.

Mentally, I was just barely holding on. Embracing a covert victim mentality, stealthily hidden, I had employed self-imposed limitations. Spiritually, I was trying all of the trending "Woo" sparkly rocks and incantations, and never feeling further away from Source and God.

I was a hot mess.

Standing on the top of a snowboard park, and not realizing what I was saying, the following words came out, "I'm so exhausted from the pressures I'm placing on myself in life. I just need a break." Taking a big air jump on my board, I hit the snow and promptly broke both my ankles.

Literally, I got what I asked for.

I've always been able to generate "coincidences," but breaking my ankles was way over the top. Frequently in my life, I would bump into old friends I was just talking about. Answering the phone before it rang. Finding things that I didn't know were lost. Generating a solution to a problem as it is emerging. Discovering symbols and novelties to reinforce a point I was making.

This "break" was ironically on target.

I've always felt that I was good at "making things happen." But after inadvertently manifesting a "break," this experience clearly changed the trajectory of my life and I needed to understand the real process that was occurring.

I began to deeply question which Universal laws were at play here.

Not having an answer yet, my logic was this—since I had called "the break" into my life, I knew I could call in "the healing." The prognosis for my recovery from the doctors and the medical world was grim. Determined to take matters into my own hands, I decided that if I could break my ankles, *I could heal them.* Surmising if I could damage the tissues, I could rebuild the tissues and make them whole again.

I didn't know how I was going to do it, but I knew it was within the power of my mind to fix what was broken.

This is when Hot Yoga entered my life. Reading the cover of a weekly newspaper in my hometown, I saw an ad that said "Hot Yoga, Make your Body Smile, $10/10 days." Since I was looking for a physical activity that I could do with the injuries I had sustained, I tore out the offer and headed down to the Yoga studio next to the river.

It was evident to me in the first class I took that the human body and the mind have the power to heal themselves, and Yoga was going to help cultivate that. I was all in. It was an excruciatingly slow practice compared to the thrill-seeking and adrenaline rush I felt as a professional snowboarder. Yet, it was exciting to begin feeling more aligned with myself.

Quickly, my physical body got stronger in all the right ways and the healing began. Within a month, I forgot the antianxiety medication and no longer took the endless pills. Once my thinking cleared and my intellect strengthened, *I felt a deepening connection to the Universe and Spirit.*

Much of my daily time and Yoga was focused on healing my ankles by simply allowing the healing to happen at the pace that ankles heal. Having the "break" and experiencing the healing was a game changer for my life. At once, I began to use the evidence of intentional manifestation for other outcomes.

Why not set and manifest wild audacious goals in all areas of my life? Going *within*, I used these expanding insights to attract ideal relationships, improve my financial state, and make bold moves in my career path. Essentially, I wanted to easily and effortlessly do all of the things that my heart desires. *This recognition placed in my heart…*

…that the universe gives us what we ask for.

The more time spent on my Yoga mat, the clearer I got about what would fulfill my preferences for my life and the desires of my personality.

Using my mind's eye and imagining what I want, I spent dedicated time asking for the things I desire. It's vital to me that whatever I ask for contributes to a better life for me and all the people I care for.

The influences of outside forces melt away with every Yoga posture I experience. The paths to daily preferences and my wildest lifelong dreams reveal themselves with every Savasana taken at the end of each Yoga session. Sometimes *within* my Yoga practice, the experience of receiving some future desire emerges from deep inside my imagination.

Often, I surface from the deep concentration on my breath during Yoga with a solution to a problem I didn't know I had. It's as if I'm enveloped in the knowledge that I am co-creating my life with Source and God. Prayer is co-creation with God for the religious. Manifestation is co-creation with Source for the rest.

Having a yoga practice has done so much for me. The method of the 26 & 2 Hot Yoga Sequence is a tool I use to take deep personal responsibility to heal, maintain, and create my life on all levels: Physically, Emotionally, Mentally, and Spiritually.

Because I now feel good, well, amazing, I am no longer running triage for a beat-up and damaged neglected self. I can connect with my desires and allow my imagination to generate the feeling of obtaining the next thing that I want from life.

By maintaining my life with my Yoga practice, I'm better able to consciously create the life I want to live.

A Yoga practice can also help you come to know your deepest desires to manifest your life's dreams and know that it will work for you. Yoga affords you the solitude to hear the whispers of your wildest dreams. This space will help you connect with Spirit and provide the clarity to see the path revealed to you to make your dreams come true.

When you're creating your life, you have the freedom to not only create but also the freedom to undo what you don't like. Literally, you have the power to either reverse the trajectory you are on or infuse your life with expanded energy that you enjoy and love. All of this can come through your heart and your thoughts.

If you're not doing so now, what would happen if you used your power to create your own fulfilling life? It's possible to truly develop a deep self-worth that provides better health, increased joy, and unbinding wonder. At the deepest level, when each of us takes care of ourselves, it is a service, not only to those that are closest to us but also a service to the world.

My 3 Tips for You:

1. **Nobody gets this far unscathed. So, begin where you are.** There is a life you'd like to live, and it can be *created*.

2. If you are sick or injured, mentally, physically, emotionally, or spiritually, **practice yoga for the other 95% of your body/being.** Give grace to the parts that need healing and keep the rest in condition. Be in shape for when you are healed.

3. Talk to yourself in the mirror like you would **to your very best friend**. Most of the things we have the nerve to say to ourselves, we wouldn't say to our worst enemies. So, be impeccable with your words.

Who's Mica?

Mica Michele Fish practices the art of co-creation, manifestation and prayer to intentionally craft the physical world as it presents itself into balance in body, mind, and spirit. She's a Creative Entrepreneur and Certified Coach with a passion for Yoga and Creating the world she wants to live in. You can find her in her backyard, Teaching Yoga in her Boutique Private Yoga studio, or playing and interplaying with nature, on her land, with the love of her life, three bonus children and a Moody Bernedoodle

To learn more about Mica Fish and all the co-authors, visit www.innerpointe.com.

Dr. Adam Chipiuk

Essay Fourteen

"Bring Forth All That Is Within You..."

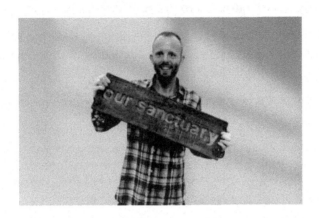

Struggling mightily during my senior year at New York University College of Dentistry, I was frustrated because I wanted to do more than fix a tooth.

Wanting to help others heal, I resented my decision to study dentistry, being bitterly disappointed that I didn't pursue medical school. My friends and colleagues were excited about graduation, opening their dental clinic, and making money to buy a big house and fancy cars but I kept repeating to myself: "What the f**k are you doing?" "Who are you?"

I knew that I was not living up to my potential and I wish I could start my life all over.

One of my favorite quotes is: *"Bring forth all that is within you... it will save you; it will save the world. If you do not bring forth all that is within you, it will destroy you; it will destroy the world." —Jesus Christ*

On the outside, I was happy, positive, and easygoing but internally, I was very angry and full of negative thoughts toward myself. I engaged in toxic behaviors, such as binge drinking, overeating, and drug use. Quickly spiraling downward, I did not recognize the man in the mirror and needed to create a massive change in my life.

"Be careful what you are thinking because all of your cells are listening."

– Emmy Cleaves

During my freshman year, a doctor lecturing said, "If you ever get cancer, Hodgkin's Lymphoma is the one to get because it has a good cure rate."

"As if you get to choose which cancer you get," I heckled.

In the darkest times, if we stand tall and hold on, the light will appear and we receive what is needed to guide us forward.

One divinely guided day, I found the courage to stare into my eyes in the mirror, I stared for hours. For several reasons, I told myself "You are going to get Hodgkin's Lymphoma."

1. I wanted to prove whether God exists...will you deliver this gift so I can restart my life?

2. If I had cancer, I would need chemotherapy, my body would waste away, and I could rebuild it from scratch. I was 40 pounds overweight because I was partying, drinking, eating too much, and could not do cardio exercises due to a recent reconstructive knee surgery.

3. If I overcome cancer, there's no obstacle or challenge in life that I couldn't find the inner strength to overcome.

A year and a half later, exactly on my 30th birthday, I was diagnosed with Hodgkin's Lymphoma. Taking a deep breath, I looked up and whispered...

"Thank you." From that point on, I realized how powerful our minds are and have focused on creating good things in life for myself and others.

During cancer treatments, I would go to the gym and work out daily (I did not yet know Yoga) because I knew cancer wasn't taking a day off from trying to kill me, so I could not take a day off from fighting it. It was now or never to live as my best version. To have the best chance of survival, I knew I needed to be my healthiest, strongest, and best self.

Finding myself physically wasting away, at one point I could only curl five-pound dumbbells. Struggling to just breathe as I ran on the treadmill, people would stare at my pale complexion and would comment because my hair was falling out. However, my mental state was incredibly strong.

Staring at myself in the mirror, I recited my mantra "F**k you, cancer, you have no idea who you are messing with." Even when my body didn't want to get up, my mind would not let me lay in bed. There was no choice but to get up, go to the gym, and try to be better than I was yesterday.

Three years later, my sister convinced me to try Bikram Yoga. From the first few breaths in Pranayama, I realized this is what I had been looking for all my life. The hot room was very humbling and eye-opening. I struggled to keep up with the other students in class. Seeing the 50–60-year-olds rocking class in the front row while I (once a top athlete) was struggling to keep up made me question what is true health and wellness. At that point, I promised myself I was going to practice Yoga for the rest of my life. Even though I was in the gym lifting weights, I was practicing Yoga without realizing it during the endless cancer treatments.

Who is the expert on health?

Do you honestly believe it is the medical doctor? Just because they wear white coats and earned an expensive degree because they studied systems and diseases. Or is the expert someone who has overcome numerous health issues and is a living example of radiant health?

Who would you rather ask for advice: an overweight, chronically ill-looking doctor, or someone that never gets sick, has no pain, doesn't take any medications, and is full of vitality?

"You're never too old, never too bad, never too late, and never too sick to start from scratch once again." When I played competitive sports, I twisted, tore, and broke many different parts of my body. If you can think of it, it happened to me. I had surgeries to repair sports injuries, chronic back pain, was significantly overweight, had depression, and was even suicidal. Before I was diagnosed with cancer, I would get terribly sick several times a year. In reality, I had a junk, broken body and mind.

But... through Yoga, I rebuilt myself from scratch.

In 2010, I began an orofacial pain and sleep residency at the University of California Los Angeles. I resigned from the program after realizing that the primary treatment offered to patients was writing prescriptions for opioids to numb them from their pain rather than healing or curing them of their illnesses. So, it was then that I enrolled in the most intense Yoga teacher training program and started over from scratch

How and why does Yoga work? Simple—Soul Power. Yoga is a scientific path towards self-realization; to take full accountability and responsibility for your health and your life; to show you who you are and the purpose of your birth.

"As above, so below, as within, so without, as the universe, so the soul." - *Hermes Trismegistus*

The 26 postures and two breathing exercises in the Bikram Yoga Method, and during the 90-minute practice, is your opportunity to see for yoursel what is and isn't working for you, not only in the Yoga room but in life During the difficult and uncomfortable moments that the postures or the hot room bring up, you learn to keep looking into your own eyes no matter how intense the struggle becomes. It is in those dark times that the answe will appear *within* for what you need to do to be better, to heal, and to thrive. The answer isn't likely what you want to do, but what you *need* to do.

Do you have the courage to do what is needed?

By looking into your own eyes, you are connecting to your Atma; you Soul, your highest self. Your soul knows what is needed to live your bes life. No one can give you the answers you are seeking because they are found *within*. The Kingdom of Heaven is *within*.

Learn to be the master of your body and mind, and watch how everything else simply falls into place.

As you practice Yoga, you learn non-attachment, to let go. By trying the postures in the right way, you are getting 100% of the benefits. The medica benefits come to you through your honest effort at that moment, not by how deep you go or how long you stay in the posture. Over the years, I've seen many students self-sabotage themselves in their practice withou realizing it.

In Yoga class, the moment the teacher says change, the posture has ended. If you think you need to stay longer to heal something then you are recreating that problem and not allowing the maximum healing benefits Just think of it: If you had no issue or problem you would start and come out of the posture when the teacher says change. No delays, no baggage no issues, no problems.

If you practice Yoga if you have no ailments, no illness, and no problems then you're an example of radiant health and wellness. When practicing from that mindset, you must believe that your body and mind have already healed and your duty is to have a consistent practice and allow the necessary time to realize this truth. Eventually, or in the future, you will create what you believe to be true in your mind.

There is one simple rule to being healthy: we invest time, energy, and money o be successful in our studies, careers, and relationships so naturally, we too must invest time, energy, and money, for our health and wellbeing. Invest more time in yourself and watch how amazingly beautiful life will unfold for you!

My 3 Tips for You…

1.Control your feet, control your life, control your destiny.

2. Never give up! If you fall out of your life or a posture, get back in. The only reason we don't reach our goals or realize our dreams is because, at some point, we decided to give up. Never give up!

3.Don't waste time and energy. Be aware, be precise, and move with intent. This is true whether you're moving about in your daily life or your Yoga practice.

Who's Dr. Adam Chipiuk?

From a young age, Adam always wanted to help others heal. Teaching yoga allows him the opportunity to inspire others to be their best version of themselves as they take ownership of their health and well-being. Adam started practicing yoga in 2010 and received his Bikram Yoga Teaching Certificate in 2011. He's taught at over 100 yoga studios around the world.

To learn more about Dr. Adam Chipiuk and all the co-authors, visit www.innerpointe.com.

BridgettAne "BA" Goddard

Essay Fifteen

"Meet Resistance with a Smile"

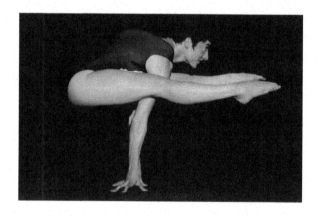

Immersed in university life at 18, and part of an extremely intensive acting program in New York, I felt the stress big time when a friend invited me to join her for a weekly Yoga class. *Both the setting and the teacher took my breath away.*

The class was offered in the chapel overlooking Lake Cayuga at sunset. Diana, our teacher, a heavily pregnant woman, made everything look easy. It blew my mind to see how she exuded such calm, inner joy, and grace while contorting her body into positions that made my head spin and muscles quiver.

From Hatha, I went on to Ashtanga but was soon disillusioned after the teacher suggested a post-class walk in the woods which resulted in him, disappointingly, crossing the line. Besides that, he said I ought to do weight training and take up cycling to acquire the necessary strength and stamina the Primary Series required. Although I was uninspired to carry on that path, I felt curious and had faith that I'd find my perfect practice.

There are so many styles of Yoga and infinite teachers in our world.

Having explored further, I dipped my toe into Vinyasa flow, but it was in 2000 when I first braved Original Hot Yoga, and from day one, I was hooked! Jimmy Barkan was my first teacher and I sat wide-eyed, spun out, nd baffled by the level of contentment in the hot room.

low was everyone seemingly so joyous?!

immy led a posture clinic after class. I stayed for hours, gobbled up tips on echnique, and bought the book and audio cassette. The next day, I caught flight back home to marry my first husband. I didn't get a chance to eturn to Yoga class until after our honeymoon.

Jnlike any other Yoga, the benefits of Hot Yoga were visible after one week is my waistband tightened. After two months, my lifelong battle with inusitis disappeared along with my acne. After six months, my low blood pressure normalized. After two years, my high cholesterol was normal; his was after being told it was hereditary and I'd be on medication for life. 'm not.

Around the same time, I began a 100-day challenge. Showing up for daily classes, I looked into the mirror and my eyes every day for three months. Eventually, I saw how sad I looked and realized how horrible I was being to myself. My teachers called it Chitta Vittri or mind chatter, but all I heard was negative self-talk. I was angry with myself for drinking the wrong drinks, eating the wrong foods, and saying yes to a marriage I knew in my heart was wrong from the moment he proposed. Georgia Balligian is one of my most influential teachers, and in the midst of my sadness, she helped me embrace a "happy, smiling face." She also suggested I show my belly, which, although difficult at first, ultimately seeing myself in the mirror allowed me to confront my real shape and realize how to properly use my muscles and reshape my body to develop more physical and emotional support.

Daily practice is the best tool to help realize what's working, what you want to maintain, what's not working, and that you have all you require to move on and let go of anything working against you.

When my teacher told me I was ready to teach, I was initially terrified, but I put my faith in her and developed more faith in myself by having Beyoncé and Destiny's Child among my first students; I couldn't refuse their request for a last-minute private session and taught subsequent one-on-one sessions with Kelly Rowland.

My biggest lesson in practicing Yoga has been to let go!

Little by little, I realize more and more how and what I can release to evolve. I let go of judgment. I let go of criticism. I let go of a desire to be the best in the room. I realized I am enough in my being the best version of myself.

Realizing my imperfections are in fact that which make me human, I soon learned to love every one of them! What used to be a trigger is now a bell of mindfulness; a gentle reminder to take time to breathe and be grateful as I notice myself.

As a Yoga teacher, my main focus is two-fold:

1. Resting in the physical to be precise in technique.

2. Inspiring folks to go to their maximum potential while realizing where less effort and less depth are more effective and beneficial (i.e., working with ailments and/or injuries).

Consider these questions and thoughts...

Are you in love with your life?

Are you your best friend and your number one fan?

You deserve to have an amazing relationship with yourself! Are you having fun?!

You are a good healer!

No matter your age or condition, if you have the desire to feel better and to live better then you have all you require to begin again. Yoga teachers may well teach you, but so much of our teaching is a reminder of what you already know *within. Quiet the voices that hold you back and simply show up and do the best you can.*

Some of the most inspiring students have suffered intense pain and trauma. Sadly, sometimes we are too comfortable to create change in our lives, but when we are desperate to get out of pain and suffering, that can be when great life changes occur. My students and teachers who choose the higher road do not get pulled into negativity, gossip, judgment, and suffering, *and who utilize darkness as an opportunity to tap into their greatest source of love and light within, are my greatest inspirations.*

My favorite Yoga books include...

The Autobiography of a Yogi by Paramahansa Yogananda

The Yoga Sutras of Patanjali by Sri Swami Satchidananda

Peace is Every Step by Thich Nhat Hanh

Rereading each one of these at different points in my life, I've found the lessons compelling to me on different levels.

What are your favorite books?

In addition to Hatha Yoga, traditional seated meditation has become a daily practice, along with Yoga Nidra before I sleep. *Yoga in the Lanes* hosts annual retreats in Spain and I am delivered to cloud nine when we have a week together of intensive training, and then able to share these daily rituals and practices with our group. We will host our second Original Hot Yoga Teacher Training in June 2023. As an ambassador of RubyMoon — gym to swim eco-wear — I lead Yoga, Breathwork, and meditation before we immerse ourselves in the cold Brighton Sea as the sunsets and the full moon rises each month. Becoming a vegetarian at age 13, a vegan at 23, and a raw foodist for six months in 2013, I have a deep love and appreciation for understanding nutrition as it became an instrumental part of my training for the International Yoga Championships.

The Yoga championships completely transformed my body, spirit, and mind. Encouraged by my teachers to first participate in 2003, I was surprised to place third in the New York State division. This led me to San Francisco and my first encounter with Mary Jarvis, an esteemed teacher, mentor, and coach to Yoga champions from all over the world. Mary encouraged me to make training part of my normal daily routine, above and beyond attending classes. "Have you done your homework?" she'd ask, and I'd say yes. "How many times?" she'd ask. I'd smile bigger and do it again. We've had so much fun together over the years and I am deeply grateful and appreciative of all the intensive training and wisdom she passes on through her teaching.

Many gravitate to Mary, as I did each year as the championships drew near. We would spend weeks together training and laughing for hours on end, culminating in my placing 11th in the world in 2013. Mary is the most generous, empowering, compassionate teacher I have known, and she's taught me many life lessons which have helped me on and off the mat. Such a great honor to be asked by her to "do it again" and again and again. We'd spend hours on Standing Bow Pulling pose alone and she helped me realize anything was possible if I was prepared to do the work and truly believe in myself.

Being diagnosed in 2008 with Interstitial Cystitis, an autoimmune disorder, my diet changed dramatically. Doctors told me I'd be on medication and in and out of the hospital for the rest of my life. Instead, I chose to do more research. I explored all options, including bioenergy healing, and to my surprise, even urine therapy.

To help heal...

I released restrictive and limiting beliefs.

I released pushing past the pain.

I no longer blamed others for my suffering.

I learned to love, respect, and appreciate my pain for the lessons it reveals

There is power in choosing light, love, wellness, and joy. As a peace bringer, I had to realize where the war was inside my body and mind This helped me recognize how powerful it is to let go of suffering and let love in. This life-long practice is fascinating, ever-evolving, humbling and empowering, and offers a worldwide network of like-minded folk moving toward a more peaceful and loving world.

My 3 Tips for You...

1. Maintain practice with a minimum of three classes per week; more often to expedite, improve, and excel.

2. Listen with your third ear and look with your third eye to release judgment, embrace imperfections, and realize your unlimited potential.

3. Practice begins where we meet resistance and easy breathing is always more important than the depth of the pose. When you lead with the breath you learn to practice with less effort and can make a challenging situation look easy, both on and off your mat. Replacing judgment, frustration, or anger with gratitude makes for efficient and effective progress.

Who's BridgettAne?

BridgettAne Goddard was born in the U.S. and raised near Chicago. She began ballet at age four, performing at five and working professionally as an actor from age 12. She began Yoga in 1995 in Ithaca, NY. Ten years later she taught Beyoncé, graduated Bikram's Teacher Training and went on to open Yoga in the Lanes in Brighton, UK. She placed 11th in the world in 2013 and is UK's head judge for the International Yoga Asana Sport Federation. Published in Yoga Magazine, "BA" continues to practice, teach and perform as an actor and lead singer for her band Atlantic Crossing.

To learn more about BridgetteAne Goddard and all the co-authors, visit www.innerpointe.com.

Donna Wikio

Essay Sixteen

"There's a crack in everything.
That's how the light gets in."
(Leonard Cohen)

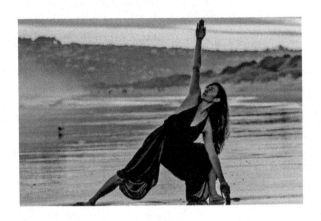

We shall start with the age-old tale of a traveler who, after years of searching and being driven to despair, finds a miraculous cure, a talisman or a wise sage to aid them, save them, and allow them to transform their existence; tales and fables abound around transformation forged in fire. When we stand in a hot yoga room, feet together nicely, looking in the mirror, things become so simple and so clear. The weight of the world falls away and the heat flushes everything out.

I sincerely feel that yoga practitioners are those modern-day travelers. We are all pressed hard against the rigidities of social expectations and technology. Crushed by the mundane realities of day-to-day existence, we wonder if there's more. Why are we here? What is even the point of it all?

A long path of searching, and perhaps longing, led me to my first Bikram Yoga class in 2005. I had practiced many other styles of Yoga and I was mostly interested in losing weight and fighting my way out of the fog of new motherhood.

I admit that initially, I was slightly disdainful of teachers that did not practice while teaching and of what seemed at first like a rigid style o yoga. Where was the chanting? Where was the incense? I would not say that I enjoyed my first class, but I could not believe how I felt walking out of the studio and into the night. I literally felt that my soul had been popped back into my body. I could feel the blood pumping through me like nothing ever had.

Not running, or saunas, or anything!

I remember thinking 'I need to do this forever.'

Fast forward a few years and I found myself both literally and figuratively at teacher training in Mexico in 2008 with a 13-month-old baby! In all honesty, I am not 100% sure how that happened, and in no way did everything fall easily into place. At the time, I was a single parent of two young children, living with my parents and really just scraping by. I was teaching multiple styles of Yoga but nothing resonated as much as the Bikram system.

Becoming a Bikram teacher, and in turn a studio owner, dramatically changed the direction of my life. New Zealand is a small country known mainly for its beauty and its many sheep! We were quite far behind the Yoga boom of the late '90s and the lower South Island in particular is known for its stoical farm folk and 'walk it off' attitude!

The decision to open up a studio in Dunedin, where I did not know anyone, was driven by the desire to settle and provide for my family and to be near the beach. Despite being the oldest city in New Zealand, it is a vibrant University town so I went with instincts rather than an amazing business plan.

It turned out that these stoical folks love yoga, and the studio has become a refuge for people from all walks of life over the past nearly 14 years!

The statistics for Maori single mothers in New Zealand are terrible, and in many ways, I have always resisted the stereotypes that had been directed at me over the years with comments like, "Well done for overcoming adversity." I believe that practicing, and in turn teaching, yoga set me on a path to success. I am university educated. My life has changed unequivocally from that first class in Wellington in 2005. My yoga studio has grown and survived the pandemic and various highs and lows in the industry at large over the last 14 years.

Loss and longing are common themes in our human existence. I found my younger sister, Kassie, dead in her crib when I was four years old and although I remember very little of the actual event, the following days haped my life in many ways.

n Maori culture, a funeral or Tangi is a fairly long affair with three days to a week of mourning.

The mourning begins at home, with the family (whanau) member in heir coffin in the lounge, and then at a Marae/Tribal meeting area for a few nights where extended family sleep together on mattresses in the Wharenui/meeting house, again with the body present. Elders of the family are always near the body, wailing, crying, and helping to assist the soul to heaven.

Last of all, the coffin is carried to a nearby Urupa (burial ground) and put to rest amongst their family. It is a very social event with shared meals and kids running around outside. It is an amazing opportunity to say goodbye to a loved one and make peace with the gods. My traumatized parents acted against their better instincts and decided it would be too much for me to attend. I was kept at home with my very loving and well-meaning Pakeha (white) maternal grandparents. Years later, when entering into relationships, I really struggled with connection; there was a deep layer of fear and mistrust that I had to spend years working through and it was only much later that I connected it to the loss of my sister and not being able to mourn her properly.

When we stand feet together looking at ourselves in the mirror, day after day, year after year, in the heat, and listen to the words of the Yoga practice, something very fundamental shifts inside.

Like a giant internal spotlight, Yoga will shine a light on all of those dark hidden things.

We can notice them, process them, and most importantly, move forward. This process, like any therapeutic practice, is not easy. It is a common idea that if the 'after Yoga' feeling could be made into a pill it would be the best-selling drug in the world.

We all want happiness; we don't want suffering and sorrow. But, without one we can never know the other. With yoga, we are given the tools to heal ourselves, free ourselves, and in turn, help others.

In my 20s, I worked as a model. While it was fun, I was never into being credited and paid for the simple genetic luck of being tall with decent bone structure. It was so exciting to become a Yoga teacher and to be in a realm where, or so I thought, everyone was healthy and happy with their bodies.

That naivety was shattered pretty fast when I realized that Yoga people are just people and the same problems and dramas exist wherever we are!

Watching with mild alarm as the wellness industry swelled in popularity over the past 10 years, I've seen many of the same old things are still there with fancy new wording. Diets are now intermittent fasts or Paleo Primal resets. Meal replacement shakes are now bone broths or collagen smoothies. We don't run to burn calories we do Peloton and eat 'clean' to live our best lives ever. Everything is designed to make us feel less than, unworthy, unfit, and body conscious.

What to do? Give up? Or just take a more cautious approach?

It is always worth stepping back and considering your source of information. If you have been eating a certain way for years and feel like crap, ask yourself why. If you have been doing a certain exercise or seeing a physio for ages and nothing is improving in terms of pain or mobility, then stop! Find another way!

You are the most important person in your life.

When looking for a Yoga practice, remember that in Yoga the longest and most thorough teacher trainings are in Iyengar, Kundalini, and Bikram, Original Hot. Never place blind faith in a teacher; ask where did they train and for how long? How is their practice? Or more importantly, do they even practice?

I like to try things and see what works. For me, fermented foods make me feel sick. I eat healthily and occasionally have a pie or fried chicken without remorse. I try to move daily, whether it's Hot Yoga, Pilates, or walking the dog.

After years of self-loathing, dieting, and eating disorders, it's pretty great to be free, but it was certainly not without struggle and effort.

Physically, Yoga has been there for me for nearly 17 years. The reasons that I came to Yoga are different from the reasons that I continue to practice. As a new Mum in her late 20s, I was experiencing the struggles of birth trauma (four days in labor), sleep deprivation, and a loss of contact or connection with my post-baby body.

Over the years, I have practiced through another pregnancy (a completely different experience and an easy birth) and two major hip surgeries, including a full hip replacement. I maintained my Yoga practice as best as I could with the deterioration of my hips due to old running injuries. When he pain became so debilitating, I struggled to walk or sleep.

Even with a hip replacement, it is amazing to be pain-free. Recovery started 10 days after my replacement, with just lying in the hot room and moving as best I could to start the process of healing. It is crucial as a teacher to let your students see you struggle, recover, and grow alongside them. I try to be open about that and in many other forms of Yoga, it is hidden away for fear of not seeming strong or flexible. In Bikram, we are all about doing the best you can with the body you have, and we promote the long goal, over any short-lived glory.

One of our greatest teachers, Emmy, may she rest in peace, said, "The only thing about this yoga is that you have to do it forever; if you stop, your body will demand that you return." Be in it for the long run; it takes commitment, but it is such a fantastic ride.

My 3 Tips for You...

1. Breathing is first, everything else is secondary.

2. Calm, normal breathing, in and out through the nose, keeps you calmer.

3. Try to let go of expectations in life and for every class.

Who's Donna?

Donna Wikio is a mum of two teenage boys and a passionate advocate of Hot Yoga as a healing modality. She can be found at her studio in Dunedin, New Zealand or tromping at the beach with her Golden Labrador! She has trained in Bikram, Ashtanga, Iyengar, Hot Pilates, Yin and Trauma Informed Yoga. In addition, she has an Honors Degree in Political Science that occasionally comes in handy at dinner parties!

To learn more about Donna Wikio and all the co-authors, visit www.innerpointe.com.

Brad Colwell

Essay Seventeen

"How to Get the Fire Started"

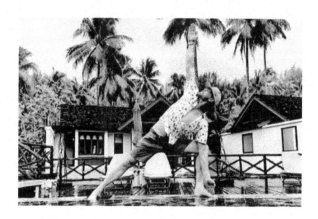

Having my own slogan for years has gone a long way but I decided to add a lead-in phrase…

How to… "Get the Fire Started"

In the fifth grade, at the ripe age of 11 years old, I seemed to note that we are all moving either from pain or to pleasure. Essentially, we all want to feel good; that somehow at the end of this life, not only were we supposed to enjoy the trip, but to feel good while doing it.

Seems simple and logical, right?

And we're off to the races. Even as a young boy, my initiative was to create 'fire' energy. Sitting around too much seemed to lack energy, so I was always 'full' of it. My mother used to call me *"fireball"* (hence my nickname starting young). I realized groups of people that would sit and read were smart and full of info but didn't have that *umph of energy* I was attracted to and craved.

Did you have a nickname growing up?

Exercise, as we all know, is good for us, physically and mentally, but there are so many types and I guess the quest of life is, which one is for me?

When I was very young, I started skating at three and played hockey at five years old. Growing up in Canada, playing hockey was an integral part of my childhood and teenage years. It was at the age of 14 when I already had my second concussion in hockey and mom clearly pronounced—as I was waking up from my second knockout—"There's no more hockey for you."

So, my continual journey of searching for an energy 'outlet' led me to downhill skiing, track and field, and running (fewer contact sports). But my real passion was motorcycle/motocross racing.

When was it in your life that you found your passion?

As I got older, as an athlete, I quickly understood the benefits of Yoga elevating the player and maintaining the play at a high level. Progress into the years of actually teaching Yoga, the avenue of teaching professional athletes was natural, giving them the edge and preparation for their game.

My students became NHL, NFL, and NBA players (without name-dropping). Once a professional player feels the effects of how the practice of Yoga elevates their game, it essentially becomes mandatory for both their physical and mental game. Kareem Abdul Jabber has claimed that Yoga kept him playing for years injury free.

From my first Yoga class in December 1999, I had absolutely no idea about it or how my life was going to change so drastically. "Oh ya, Yoga, it's stretching, right?"

Do I need to be religious? Nope!

It became increasingly important to ensure I was moving in the direction of health, wellness, and longevity. When I started teaching Yoga in late 2000, it sunk in that hot Yoga hits all three categories of self-satisfaction—*mental, physical, and spiritual.*

What preconception did you have about Yoga?

Needless to say, after 90 minutes of the most remarkable and sweaty Yoga class, I came out and plunked myself onto the wooden bench, and literally watched a light bulb come on over my head (like a cartoon) and I said to myself… **"I'll be doing this for the rest of my life."**

Have you ever had that bright insight sensation before?

Now, I didn't say or even consider that I would be a Yoga teacher or one day an owner of a thriving Yoga school, but that new incredible sense of well-being was at its highest peak and it was clear that I had finally found my thing! What I didn't get (yet), was that I started making a profound connection with myself; it felt like a whole new level of personal awareness that I never knew was there.

About six months in was when I was asked by my Yoga teacher to go to teacher training, even though I felt I had no knowledge of this ancient Yoga practice.

"How could I possibly teach Yoga?"

Needless to say, after an intense nine-week teacher training, I discovered a phenomenal new skip to my step. From there, I felt destined to encourage, influence, and promote Yoga to as many people as I could.

"Why would anyone do Yoga?"

[my answer] *I don't know, maybe to feel good!* And then my other friend pipes in and says, "I can drink a beer and feel good, why would I do Yoga?"

Good question and the hard right answer is, "You never know how it feels until you go into class." When I get asked on the street or in a coffee shop, "What will I get from Yoga?" my answer simply is, ***"It's like I'm about to give you a piece of gold; it's in my hand, but the only way you get the gold is by showing up, and having your own experience. Once someone 'feels the gold' they, too, have their right answer."***

After owning/operating and teaching at my own Yoga school in Vancouver, British Columbia for 11 years, I was invited by global Yoga studios to come to teach and demonstrate what I had learned (on the business side as well). Traveling internationally taught me that no matter where you came from, any level of fitness and any injury could be overcome by consistent Yoga practice. I started doing laps around the blue marble and the conclusion was clear—this was an international regime that virtually everyone could benefit from.

My second favorite quote is: *"THE HARDEST PART IS SHOWING UP!"*

Injuries are a big part of life, physically and mentally, so the fact that the ancient art of Yoga helps repair, fix, and heal chronic long-term pain was and is a big motivator for me.

When I started my Yoga journey, I suffered endless bouts of long-term chronic back pain. I used to race motocross motorcycles from ages 10-20; I was even sponsored by Honda and Yamaha.

After performing countless 50ft jumps in the air on my bike, my spine

ecame like an accordion. By 20 years old, walking had become extremely
ifficult. I spent the ages 20-30 going to a chiropractor three times a week,
vith a huge dose of massage therapy and acupuncture.

)nce I hit 30 years old, I thought managing endless pain in my body was
/hat I would have to live with for the rest of my life. Day after day, it often
ecame impossible to get out of bed. The fear set in that I could literally be
rippled for life.

o then came Yoga, and I felt immediate relief!

everal X-rays of my spine showed massive compression and deterioration
f the lower discs in my lumbar spine. The doctors claimed that it simply
vasn't repairable.

But then how could I feel so good doing this Yoga?" My body literally needed
) relearn how to

tand straight.

itting straight, without slouching, became my daily mantra.

ven bending over to pick up a box with ease had to be discovered all over
gain. It took a few years to tear down all that scar tissue that was built up
) 'protect' my back. Countless Yoga classes helped to rebuild soft tissue
nd muscle around the spine, which helped to support my back so it could
love fluidly without pain. This is truly where I learned about Yoga, about
lyself, my belief system, and who I really was. Not only was I unwinding
le pain in my body, but I was also relearning about myself through the
lirror of my own eyes.

*f you are experiencing any level of chronic pain, do everything you can to get to a
ot Yoga class. With regular practice, you'll find the path to let it go.*

\ Yoga journey can take you to personal depths *within* that can barely be
xplained with words. For anything to truly get better, it will often get
vorse before it improves. Having been there and done that is why today, I
an offer deep confidence to anyone that requires repair.

'he spiritual part of Yoga was now coming into my existence. We all have
eard the word spiritual but the words of my experience through my
eacher came clear: ***"To truly know thyself."***

'hrough my journey of healing, connecting, understanding myself, and
eeling effing phenomenal all the time, I can now be super motivational
） start encouraging others at a high-speed rate and shout through a

megaphone, *"EVERYONE NEEDS TO BE DOING YOGA!!"* Anyone that shows up to class and practices regularly will help take their life to the next level. Why? *Because Yoga works.*

Welcome…let's get the fire started!

My 3 Tips for You…

1. For your first yoga class, have zero expectations of what it is, and approach it by focusing on your breath the entire class (put less focus on the postures).

2. Drink water (and electrolytes) all day and before class! If you're thirsty in class, it's too late. This helps you immensely!

3. Showing up for anything is a difficult motivation. Bring a friend, neighbor, or relative and mutually support each other.

Who's Brad?

Brad Colwell is a super passionate yogi devoted to helping humanity through his personal healing experiences. His Yoga journey since 2000, has had him owning and operating multiple studios in Canada and the U.S. Due to his strong addiction to health and well-being, he keeps a busy schedule traveling the world teaching classes and training new Yoga teachers.

To learn more about Brad Colwell and all the co-authors, visit www.innerpointe.com.

Danelle Denstone

Essay Eighteen

"Quality of Life for the Rest of Your Life"

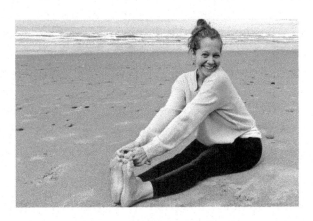

Emotionally, I felt empty and lost. There were so many days that it was difficult for me to function in the way that I wanted. It often seemed as if I was very disconnected from myself and didn't know how to get out of it. It was 1999 and I was working in operations for Southwest Airlines in San Diego.

At 26 years old, I would work 17 hours a day for 10 days straight, then with my free tickets, I would travel all over the world. Immersing myself in my travels and experiencing new and exciting cultures was very fulfilling, but in other ways, it was an escape from facing things I needed to face.

Africa and the Greek Islands were among my favorite destinations. Even while I would marvel at the sights and remark on what a contrast it was from what I knew back home, there was something else I kept looking for in my travels. I was looking for understanding. I would study the people and try to understand their culture, in hopes of understanding myself more deeply. I tried to see myself in them—in the faces of the people I saw.

Back home, I started exploring my underlying emotional pain. For eight years, I had been diving into my pain with a therapist. It was great to talk and get everything out, yet I really wanted to just get past it all and heal.

Many of my friends were encouraging me to try this thing called Bikram

Yoga. The wild stories I kept hearing about the heat and sweating seemed unreal. Really? You go to Yoga in a heated room and sweat?

Yet, they always seemed so happy and joyful—they were glowing and smiling all the time.

A colleague kept nudging me to give it a try and gifted me a 5-class card to help me get my foot in the door. I took the plunge, and I couldn't believe it: Dick Smothers (the comedian) was waiting at the front door to go into the Yoga class. He seemed excited to tell me all about it and how much he loved Bikram Yoga.

As we were finding our spots and settling in, I caught a glimpse of Mr. Smothers in his little black Speedo! Now, I really was laughing inside to myself. "What had I gotten myself into?" I thought. Soon enough, the class was underway. Even though I fumbled a bit moving through class, the teacher was very encouraging and before I knew it, 90 minutes had passed.

I never felt such bliss!!

Immediately, I was hooked! I just knew deep within that Bikram Yoga was just the thing I needed to heal myself.

Shortly thereafter, I moved to Portland and…

…the first thing I did was look for a studio. From my very first ascent up the stairs, little did I know, I found the place I would grow up in and one day call my own: Bikram Yoga Fremont Street.

It was not an easy beginning. It wasn't the physical part for me that was so hard, but once I started getting deeper into the postures, I soon realized it was the emotional part that was difficult. And that part is not always obvious on the outside. I cried a lot, I almost quit many times, I beat myself up, but I knew I needed this!

The teachers can help align your body due to injuries, but when it's your emotions, it's all on you, looking at yourself in the mirror and learning how to love what you see.

My Yoga practice brought to the surface all the emotions that were stored in my body and that is how I truly began to heal myself. Over the years, I gradually got stronger mentally and emotionally. Thankfully, in my 13th year, there was a turning point. The struggle lifted. There suddenly became a true ease to my practice and it became more meditative.

have never stopped practicing in over 20 years. Even while I was pregnant with my son, Ethan, I practiced three times a week, until the day he was born. I took three weeks off after his birth before I returned to the hot room. Yoga has become a way of life for me; it's the consistency of months and years I count on, not just days. Now, I feel my best when I practice five or six times a week.

Emmy Cleaves was my first inspirational teacher. She was 77 when I went to training. I will never forget the way she held herself at her age. She was always so alive and walked with such confidence and ease. Emmy told us about how she had some diagnostic tests performed by the doctors, and the tests revealed that all her organs were functioning as if she was in her 50s. This inspired me so much to want to maintain my health as long as possible.

I just knew I wanted to achieve what she had!

In 2006, I dove into becoming a Yoga teacher. It was also the same year I graduated from massage school. I distinctly remember some of my fellow massage students being very skeptical about how much back bending we did in Yoga.

"Once you reach a certain age you should not do backbends," they said. "Backbends are not what makes a strong spine, it is crunches," was something else they said. What!!?? I was speechless. This fueled my curiosity and my need to understand the spine and why back bending is so good for us.

One of the most important aspects of Yoga is back bending. When we bend our spine backward, we contract all the muscles along the spine. This strengthens the muscles and prevents our vertebrae from misalignment, which can lead to pressure on a nerve causing its function to decrease.

Having a structurally strong spine also protects our spinal cord. Our spinal cord is the central throughway of information and carries signals to the brain that controls everything from how we move our body to what hormones are released in order to maintain homeostasis.

The health of our spine is vital to the health of many of our systems, including the digestive system, endocrine system, immune system, and more.

Back bending counters all the forward bending we do. In our normal daily activities, we do so much forward bending, from driving, sitting, eating, working, etc. This puts pressure on our discs and lengthens our spinal muscles, which over time can weaken them, and reduce the integrity and strength of the spine. It is rare that in our activities we bend our spine backwards.

Our Yoga series does just that! Every single class, every single time. After years and years, and with consistency, the spine becomes so strong.

"The spine is the source of all energy in human life. Healthy spine, healthy life." – Bishnu Ghosh

Shifting from a teacher to a studio owner and being of service has been one of the biggest gifts in my lifetime. The advantage of knowing many of my students for decades allows me the opportunity to see the positive impact a lifelong practice can have! People tell me their stories every day; their bodies heal, and their lives change, and I get to be a part of that! It's such a blessing. The testimonies range from reducing medications, healing after disease, less pain, canceling surgeries, and more. Overall, their quality of life improves significantly.

Quality of life, for the rest of your life.

Yoga is defined as "union." The goal of Yoga is self-realization. It is a union of our soul with our higher soul; freeing ourselves from illusions, so that we can understand the truth of reality, and the truth of who we are. This is self-realization to me.

Regular Yoga practice has prepared me for much deeper work, Kriya Yoga. I began to practice Kriya Yoga, the meditation techniques and teachings of Paramahansa Yogananda, in 2020. My first introduction to the Indian-born mystic, Paramahansa Yogananda, was where I used to walk the beautiful meditation gardens of the Self-Realization Fellowship in Encinitas, CA overlooking the Pacific Ocean. The grounds are a remarkable sanctuary of tranquility. Being there brought me so much peace during a turbulent time in my life. The connection that he was the brother of Bikram Choudhury's guru, Bishnu Ghosh, didn't occur to me until many years later. No wonder the Kriya Yoga practice had been calling out to me for so many years.

It is in meditation that I truly find the meaning of self-realization.

However, it is because of my Bikram Yoga practice that I have healed my physical, mental, and emotional body—the first step in my healing process. The strength of my spine and body makes it possible for me to sit in meditation for many hours at a time. I see now that the past 20 years have been preparation for the best and final part of my healing journey, which is spiritual.

My 3 Tips for You...

1. Be proud of yourself. It takes courage to show up.

2. Strive for consistency.

3. It's best to do 1% of the posture in correct alignment and grow from here.

Who's Danelle?

Danelle Denstone's energy is high, yet you will feel her passion for Yoga. She has a calming presence that will instantly put you at ease. During her class, Danelle brings all her experiences to her teaching style. As she guides you, you will find the meditation becomes pronounced, allowing you to discover for yourself, all the great things you are capable of.

To learn more about Danelle Denstone and all the co-authors, visit www.innerpointe.com

Judy Louie

Essay Nineteen

"Living Your Dream"

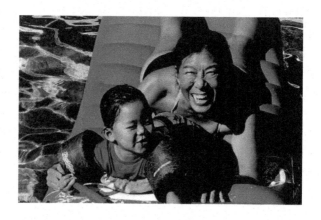

In 1995, while on vacation in Key West, Florida, my journey to becoming a yoga teacher started with a simple invitation to try a hot Yoga class. Other than one yoga class at the local YMCA, this was my first real introduction to the transformative powers of the practice.

Despite the challenge of the 90-minute class in a heated room, I was immediately hooked by how alive and exhilarated I felt after the class. When I returned home to New York, I searched for Bikram Yoga classes but couldn't find one in the early days of the practice. When I inquired at a local yoga studio about hot yoga, I was told it was nothing but a fad. Despite the feedback, this amazing yoga had given me just the vigor and passion I needed in my life and…

…I wasn't going to let it go.

A few months passed and I went on a trip back to my hometown of Portland, Oregon. I told my friend about this Yoga and she said there was a studio in Portland, and that Bikram himself would be coming to town to recruit people for his teacher training program. I couldn't believe it! I was so excited and knew this was my calling.

I couldn't believe the synchronicity.

Despite the cost, I felt compelled to pursue my newfound passion for Yoga. I sold my car and signed up for the training program. I had been working in menial jobs with no real aspirations, but now that I found yoga, I wanted to learn all I could; it literally saved my life!

There was skepticism about my decision from some, including my own mother, and they questioned why I was giving this "guy" my money. Letting the negative opinions of others deter me was not part of who I was. Deep down *within*, Yoga was my calling. Regardless, I threw myself into the teacher training with all my heart. Remember, this was 1995 when Yoga was still starting to emerge in the West.

After completing the training in Los Angeles, I returned to my hometown of Portland and immediately started to teach. It is a common belief that, with determination and hard work, anything can be achieved. As a Bikram Yoga instructor, I followed my passion against the odds.

The thirst for all forms of Yoga did not stop there. Pouring myself in, I practiced and studied many forms of yoga, including Yin Yoga, Ashtanga Yoga, Power Yoga, Anusara Yoga, and Forest Yoga. I loved it all and my practice and teaching were infused with this knowledge.

There is a Chinese Proverb that has been my compass:

"There are many paths that lead to the top of the Mountain."

In 1999, I moved to Kauai to teach Bikram Yoga at Yoga Hanalei with Lynn Moffett, one of the owners. I'm grateful to Lynn for giving me the opportunity to teach and live on the beautiful island of Kauai.

About a year later, I opened my own studio, Bikram Yoga Kauai, in Kapaa. The studio was a community hub for Yoga, dance, music, massage, and many other modalities of expression. I loved the studio and all the people that came through the doors. Quickly, I started hosting Yoga retreats to Hawaii and loved creating a safe space—a place where students could come for a week and experience practicing Yoga daily, eating island-grown food, and exploring the magic of the islands.

Yoga has given me so much and has been a testament to believing in myself and the focus it cultivates from regular practice. My journey with wanting to be a mother later in life has been a challenge, but the years of regular practice have helped bring out the courage, determination, and perseverance that were always *within*.

After years of failed attempts to get pregnant, I was determined to find another way. But, at 54 years old, there were not a lot of other options. My partner was waning with the prospect of being a parent, especially since we were now in our 50s. However, I did not want to give up my dream of becoming a mother and caring for my child. Although the odds were against me, I was very determined and focused.

I feel the years of dedicated practice prepared my body and mind to achieve the impossible. At 54, I became pregnant through IVF and gave birth at 55! My body did not fail me, and my mind gave me the strength and confidence that I needed. Yoga highlights the transformative power of practice, not just as a physical exercise, but as a mental practice where you can train and harness the power of the mind.

Pregnancy was a transformative experience that deepened my appreciation and understanding of the benefits of yoga. When I became pregnant, I was, of course, overjoyed! With the normal changes during pregnancy, I continued to practice in a modified way. It was an instrumental way to navigate the physical and emotional changes that were occurring in my body.

As the pregnancy progressed, I began to experience the profound impact that Yoga had on my emotional well-being. I found that my practice helped me to cultivate a sense of calm and acceptance, even in the face of the unknown and unpredictable aspects of pregnancy and childbirth. I attribute the deeper connection that I felt to my body and my growing baby to the mindfulness and awareness that Yoga cultivates.

Being pregnant was a total joy!

After giving birth, I continued to practice yoga as a way to support my physical recovery and mental well-being. All the breathing techniques and postures helped me to rebuild strength and energy, while also providing a sense of grounding and balance in the midst of the demands of early motherhood.

Having a child at 55 is not for everyone, and many may think I am crazy. However, this was my journey and I couldn't be more grateful. The wisdom, resources, and consciousness of being older have made me a better parent. It has been an asset as I raise my child with more patience and awareness.

I realize it is not for everyone to have a child so late in life, but it is possible. Being a mother has enriched my life in countless ways, especially as I continue on this spiritual path where my son is now a profound teacher in my life. My story is a testament to the power of following your dreams, even when others doubt you or when the path ahead seems uncertain.

I believe that anyone can achieve their goals if they are willing to focus on their intention and believe in themselves.

As a longtime Yoga teacher, I have seen firsthand how Yoga can transform people's lives. I believe that the practice can help people connect with their bodies and minds, reduce stress and anxiety, and cultivate a sense of inner peace and calm.

My 3 Tips for You...

1. Start where you are: It's easy to get intimidated by the seemingly perfect bodies and advanced poses you see on social media or in Yoga classes. But the truth is, everyone starts somewhere. Don't be afraid to take a beginner's class or modify poses to suit your body's needs.

2. Be patient: Yoga is not a quick fix. It takes time and dedication to see results. Don't get discouraged if you don't see progress right away. Keep showing up and the benefits will come.

3. Listen to your body: Yoga is not a competition. It's about tuning in to your body's needs and honoring them. If a pose doesn't feel right, don't force it. Your body knows best, so trust its wisdom.

Who's Judy?

Judy Louie has a deep passion for Yoga which has led her down a path that has transformed not only her own life but the lives of countless others. She hopes to inspire as many people as possible to pursue their dreams and live their best lives ever. Since 1995, Judy has taught Yoga as much as possible, including conducting regular retreats in Hawaii and Mexico.

For more information about Judy Louie and other authors, visit www.innerpointe.com

Bynay Blasberg

Essay Twenty

"Grow Through What You Go Through"

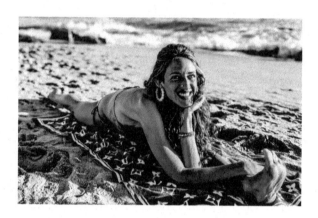

At only 15 years old, no one could have predicted the unconventional path I was about to take in life. When I officially withdrew from high school, it was evident that I would not follow the typical route.

While I had many friends, I never felt a sense of belonging.

Always being perceived as the one who marched to the beat of their own drum, I couldn't help but feel the weight of others' opinions. It was as if I had a switch inside of me that allowed me to feel what others were feeling and see their thoughts just by looking into their eyes. I was different, and everyone knew it. Those who couldn't accept it pretended to.

I wouldn't say I liked the superficiality and phoniness of people. However, I found solace in team sports, which allowed me to deal with my psychological burden of feeling people's feelings because it gave me control of that switch. I loved feeling the intense pressure and extreme discipline of basketball as we went undefeated.

Growing up in the footsteps of my older sisters, who played basketball and volleyball, I excelled in cross country, track, basketball, and soccer. After entering high school in Tucson, Arizona, I joined the women's basketball team, which General Patton's granddaughter coached. Our team was also blessed to have Lute Olsen's grandchildren playing on varsity.

The love for doing hard work that I don't always want to do but persevere anyway has been an attitude that I learned to foster.

And, the day I withdrew from high school, nothing stayed the same.

College became my new challenge, and I needed a new outlet physically. My good friend, Heather, introduced me to Bikram Yoga, and from the moment I entered that hot room, I knew my life was about to be different. I had no idea what I was getting myself into, but I was hooked from the first class.

At first, I didn't realize that my journey into Yoga would be the beginning of a transformative relationship with myself. As I gazed into the mirrored walls, I discovered I had never learned to appreciate my body. My parents believed in tough love, so self-love and acceptance were not necessarily on their radar. In my family of six, approval determined my identity. Frustrated with the roll of skin or layer of fat that stretched across my muscles every time I bent into a Yoga posture, I felt torn apart by my perception of my body.

As a former athlete, I had never seen myself in such a raw, exposed state.

Bikram yoga challenged me in ways I never expected. Despite being in excellent cardiovascular shape, I found the ninety-minute sessions torturous. The first breathing exercise, 26 postures, and the last breathing exercise were simple but extremely complex. I couldn't understand what was so tricky about them, but I kept returning for more. Every class presented new challenges and kept me intrigued.

My teacher, Bob, saw my potential and wanted me to be his first teacher employee, but my parents disapproved.

As someone who had been an athlete all their life, I knew my body well. However, this sequence of postures showed me there was much more to learn. The 90-minute torture chamber was brutal, and I struggled to breathe appropriately, despite my excellent cardiovascular shape.

It wasn't until later that I learned the principles of breathing intentionally and the importance of strengthening the muscles that support breathing. Yoga can auto-inform the body about the external environment, passing information through the peripheral nervous system to the central nervous system. I had never considered that breath control was a critical part of the practice. Now, I can't imagine practicing without it.

In 2011, I decided to attend the nine-week teacher training in Los Angeles.

Little did I know that this decision would lead to a complete transformation of my health and my outlook on life. The training was grueling, but I was determined to see it through. Unfortunately, despite my 11 years of experience, I struggled through the workouts, throwing up frequently in class for the first three weeks.

Then, in 2013, I was diagnosed with breast cancer. I had planned to undergo chemotherapy, but a close friend and fellow teacher changed my life with her advice. She told me that I shouldn't do it if I didn't believe in chemo.

So, I made a radical change in my lifestyle instead.

The sun glistened off the waves as I made my way to Bikram Yoga in Laguna Beach. It had been my home-away-from-home studio for years. Moving to Laguna was a dream come true and I went right back to the community where this yoga had been my saving grace. Later, in the summer of 2022, I found a weird lump in my left armpit. A rare form of cancer was diagnosed, and I had to undergo surgery to remove the tumor and replace old implants. A nightmare of infection, pain, and six surgeries in less than nine months left me without both breasts.

Also, underneath the left implant, something even more sinister lurked — the tumor was never entirely removed, and what was left of it migrated, quietly growing in the empty socket of my left breast. What followed was a nightmare of infection, pain, and a failed healing process that left me without both implants.

Refusing chemo and radiation, I returned to the hot room, the sanctuary where I rebuilt my strength from the ground up.

Yoga showed me that I can always grow no matter what I go through.

Teaching yoga had been my passion for years, and I knew firsthand how it could help heal the body and mind. Yoga became my lifeline as I fought through surgeries and sought to heal myself. I didn't just attend the classes — I immersed myself in the Yoga community, participating in every masterclass and clinic that top practitioners and teachers hosted. Every time I went to yoga, I felt the sparks of power and healing light inside me.

As an individual relentlessly pursuing a healthy body, I believed I had everything under control.

However, my confidence shattered when I was hit with a sudden second cancer diagnosis. In my quest for answers, I uncovered a concerning truth — society, particularly the US, fails to comprehend the complexity of diseases. Instead, our medical model prioritizes diagnosing and treating symptoms, dismissing the crucial investigation into the root causes of cellular disruption, separating the mind from the physical body, and dismissing the impacts of emotions on health. The Western model breaks the body into its parts and functions and does not value the holistic view of the body as an organism.

Yet, the more I delved, the clearer it became that finding a tangible health model was a daunting task. The institutions that claim to inform us about health and its definition were under the patronage of the same entities sponsoring the majority of academic curriculums, including those within the non-medical fields. To my dismay, these sponsors turned out to be colossal conglomerates composed of agricultural companies, tech firms, and pharmaceutical corporations that heavily influenced the information we received on health.

I was in an environment with no model for health, happiness, and healing.

I learned the hard way that preventive health action was inconvenient and impractical. The FDA, the body responsible for setting health and safety regulations for drug-grade chemicals and food, imposed numerous rules and regulations on preventative healthcare.

Through these specific 26 postures and two breathing exercises, I worked to reboot my immune system and rebuild my cellular function from the ground up. While I may be left without breasts, I have gained a deep understanding of the struggle many others face.

Despite all these challenges, Bikram Yoga is the most comprehensive solution for cellular exchange and repairing challenging health conditions. Having a reliable and consistent practice sustained me through it all.

It has not been an easy journey, but I am reminded every day that the body and mind are capable of incredible things, especially when we have the courage to grow through what we go through.

As I finally emerged cancer-free, I knew that my journey had given me a profound understanding of the human capacity for resilience and transformation.

And for that, I am grateful.

My 3 Tips for You...

1. **Form:** Precise therapeutic movements are the foundation for bodily realignment, rewiring, and recalibration.

2. **Function:** The physiological processes involved in establishing proper physical form are diverse and include building strength, increasing flexibility, improving cellular redox reactions, and enhancing myofascial neuroplasticity, resulting in various outcomes.

3. **Finesse:** Combines form and function to create a harmonic flow that results in effortless ease while using intentional breath control.

Who's Bynay?

Bynay Blosberg is a human potential coach, lifestyle mentor and Yoga teacher. Her ultimate goal is to help people flourish in life, regardless of their past struggles. Bynay specializes in assisting individuals in identifying and resolving emotional baggage and traumas, breaking free from past beliefs and behaviors, and creating a life filled with purpose and zeal. Whether you're a newcomer to self-discovery or have struggled with mental health issues before, Bynay can help walk you through your personal journey to uncover the barriers holding you back.

To learn more about Bynay Blosberg and all the co-authors, visit www.innerpointe.com.

Angelica & Zeb

Essay Twenty-One

"Save the Humans"

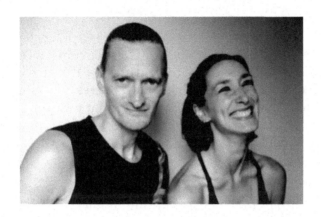

started as a funny T-shirt... "Save the Humans," kind of like that old ~ave the Whales" campaign from the '80s which helped raise awareness ~out how they were in danger. Well, guess who's in danger now?

~ you saw that on the street, "Save the Humans," would it make you stop ~nd think? Laugh? Cry?

~s a bit of a tall order, isn't it? It's pretty bold to assume that just by ~aching yoga classes anyone could "Save the Humans" from their egos, ~eir poor physical health, their mental problems, or their spiritual unrest. ~ut despite its tongue-in-cheek origins, it is our mission. We believe in yoga ~ a vehicle for service, one that invites individuals called to step onto their ~ats to find their true nature. This is the brilliance of being on the yogic ~ath: the journey back to SELF.

~ach person has *within* themselves the means to heal their body, mind, and ~irit through a consistent practice of yoga on and off the mat. But having ~e ability doesn't mean anything if you don't know how to use it. Most ~ us don't have the training, knowledge, or self-discipline to practice solo. ~racticing yoga as a lifelong discipline is enriched through having teachers, ~entors, and guides. We are grateful to have had the wisdom and support ~ many teachers and mentors from whom we are passing the teachings ~ our students. Our entrepreneurial spirits have been intertwined to give that gift back by enhancing yoga as an industry, in an iconic steel-town spirit.

"Funny name, Yoga Factory..."

Part of it comes from our roots in Pittsburgh, and part of it from the industrial building we made our home. Just like in a factory, it takes many parts to create a whole. Our "production" process incorporates multiple educational modalities that have come together under one combined vision to "Save the Humans."

Coming to our yoga practices through different circumstances, the crossing of our paths was serendipitous. Yoga can serve the greater community when delivered through the right channels: classes, workshops, trainings, retreats, continuing education, and wellness programs. Yoga, as the ancient teachings say, is a path of service. This aspect of service brought us together and helped us develop our schools, and our offerings, to Pittsburgh and beyond.

Zeb: Even as a young child, I remember doing postures out of a book and chanting "om" around the house with my mother. I was a soccer player and a runner, then attended college to pursue theater arts. After several years of traveling to major cities, I landed in San Francisco, thinking to start a life there with a couple of high school friends. I ended up with a front desk job at a nearby studio that was hiring, and within just a few classes I knew this was what I needed to do. Everything immediately clicked; recognized that transformation was imminent. A simple desk job became a fierce passion. I had to impatiently wait for my teachers to let me go to training after a mere eight months, but finally went, and continued training for years with world-renowned teachers. I traveled around the world in backpack, hopping from studio to studio to teach.

What a life of freedom!

That being said, I NEVER intended to return to Pittsburgh. But, the former owner of Bikram Yoga Pittsburgh "twisted my arm" and gave me a deal couldn't refuse. I knew I had a bigger calling to leadership, but owning yoga studio wasn't how I thought I would honor that. However, owning the studio, in addition to all the knowledge I gained about the yoga industry through traveling, lead to the start of Yoga Factory Teacher Training and other educational projects. That's how I met Angelica.

Angelica: I was busy managing a dance school in Baltimore and enjoying my professional dance career when I was first introduced to yoga. A college professor assigned the Original Hot Yoga as a required cross-training discipline for advanced-level dance majors. While I didn't necessarily have a choice, I also couldn't say "no" to continuing my practice on a free paid membership. I swore I would never practice yoga more than once per week; I had auditions to prepare for and dance technique classes to attend, right?

But yoga gradually filled my athletic void and allowed me to replace the 8-10 hours of daily rehearsals from my college days with something more fulfilling. After becoming friends with the Baltimore studio owners, and eventually becoming their manager, I got the itch to become an instructor. Unlike Zeb, it took me eight years (not eight months) to decide to take this step. If Zeb has taught me anything though, ironically, it's patience!

During the training, it became instantly clear that Zeb was someone I wanted to work with. He had a bigger vision and an ambition that I saw in myself as a budding entrepreneur. Just my luck, he had a full-time teaching position open at Yoga Factory. My personal life had recently crumbled, and I was intending to move anyhow, so Pittsburgh became my next destination.

Zeb: I was happy to have Angelica join the team as I was moving many parts (in the Yoga "Factory"): studio ownership, teacher trainings, retreats, and workshops. But to serve a broader segment of the community, we had to shift the Hot Yoga industry in a bigger way. The militant discipline and egoism weren't working. Being past my competition years, it was also becoming clear that yoga could not continue to be just about postures or a good workout. To better understand the origins and the meaning of yoga, I went to India, where this industry all started.

Experiencing the culture, teachings, and spirituality in India allowed me to open up to yoga as a philosophy and as a way of life. Yoga is a means of quieting the mind and became the way to reconnect with my true self. Yoga postures and sequences are powerful tools, but they are much more recent. I decided to add the teachings of yoga history and philosophy to what we already offer at Yoga Factory. It was a gradual shift and took people time to accept it, but Angelica deeply shared that belief.

Angelica: It's true! I was slowly shifting my relationship with dance, and focusing more on what movement meant to me. I had the lightbulb moment mid-pandemic that movement was my meditation and my method for understanding who I was. As Zeb and I continued to align in our respective journeys of self-study, we gradually began collaborating more on programming that provided tools for students to learn more about themselves, how deep yoga asana practices translate to life off the mat, and how the yogic path can create a rich life of meaningful experiences.

Also during this time, I came into my abilities as an intuitive. It was divine intervention that landed me in Pittsburgh, and the synchronous happenings after that were hard to ignore. After a "calling" to a graduate program in Addictions Counseling, several students began to confide in me about their struggles in recovery. Another few lightbulb moments later, it was time to shift to life on the yogic path, use my natural gifts, teach, and be of service. I wanted to understand the mind, and how to shape and reprogram it, so others could understand its true, unblemished nature.

Three years later, yoga and my studies in mental health birthed Yoga Recovery Pittsburgh. In line with Zeb's overarching vision for Yoga Factory, I used a lot of what he shared from his time in India to develop programs that instilled mindfulness, self-awareness, and self-love through asana practice, retreats, energetic healing, and wellness events.

Zeb: I always saw that spark in Angelica; she has so much to give. It wasn't long after she became a business owner that the opportunity presented itself to have her become co-owner of Yoga Factory. We were already overlapping on many projects; in order to embark on the next phase of my yogic journey and infiltrate the yoga industry on a bigger, (hopefully) international scale, I needed someone by my side. Angelica was more than capable and embodies Yoga Factory's mission. It made sense. But as they say, "When it rains, it pours." Within weeks of deciding to become co-owners, we were approached about opening a second location. I would not have entertained the idea without her, but as two eager entrepreneurs, we decided this was the next step forward.

A huge part of the philosophy that we teach rests on the idea of being in the present moment: "Be here now." That involves not getting too excited or too worried about the future (if we did, we wouldn't be where we are today). Teaching students YOGA (beyond the postures) is the ultimate goal on the yogic path, which we are still both on together.

We have learned that the more whole, complete, and connected one is with their true self, the more one can connect with others and raise the vibration of the planet. We certainly did that with each other. Our roots in the hot yoga system are a big part of what we teach, but there is a larger responsibility to honor yoga as a way of life and a discipline. Just like our teachers before us, we try to pass this along to anyone who chooses to step onto their mat.

Whether or not you practice yoga, what are you doing to look *within* to feel that connection with your true self? Can you step onto the mat and begin that journey?

f so, join us to help… *"Save the Humans."*

)ur 3 Tips for You…

. The yogic path is not linear; everyone's path will look different. Commit ɔ the present moment and embrace the journey to self-realization.

. Every soul is worthy of love. The purpose of practicing yoga is to come •ack to your true self, so you can see worthiness in yourself and everything round you.

. Yoga is a service. Dedicate yourself to serving your community through ʳoga on and off the mat: raise the collective vibration.

ᐯho's Angelica & Zeb?

Ⅎngelica Daniele (M.A., M.S., E-RYT) is the co-owner of Yoga Factory and ʳoordinates the school and retreats, trainings, and education programs. Ⅎngelica is a Reiki Master and Therapist with an independent practice as ɔart of her nonprofit, Yoga Recovery Pittsburgh. Angelica is also the owner •f Radiant Elle, a yoga clothing line.

ᒿeb Homison is the co-owner of Yoga Factory and Director of Yoga Factory ʳeacher Training. Zeb has been teaching and practicing yoga since 2007 and ₅ the 2014 International Asana Champion. He is a Level 3 teacher with the ɔriginal Hot Yoga Association and a 500 Hour E-RYT with Yoga Alliance.

ʳo learn more about Angelica & Zeb and all the co-authors, visit ᴡww.innerpointe.com.

Photo Credit: Anita Buzzy Prentiss

Amy Kreminski

Essay Twenty-Two

"Oh, The Places You Will GO"

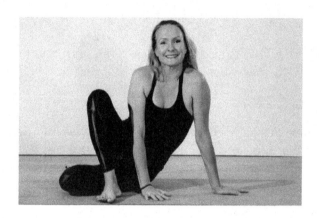

On that fateful rainy afternoon when I was walking up the hill to my first Yoga class, I never imagined where this incredible journey would lead me.

After a bitter breakup at 25 years old, with the supposed love of my life, I decided that I needed to get away from my hometown of Adelaide, South Australia. Buying myself a one-way ticket to Europe, I navigated my way from Ireland to Jersey, Channel Islands. It was there while working corporate that my days were filled in an office. After work, my time was spent in a trendy bar discussing the day's antics.

My boss drove a flashy red sports Mercedes and was someone I really admired. On the weekends, we would drive around the island going to bars, restaurants, and shopping—generally, being fabulous. France was a short ferry away and often I would head over for the day to shop or check out a new restaurant. It was often a blur as the day was filled with Champagne and chartreuse.

Then one fateful day, while dressing, I was having problems putting on my shoes. At the ripe age of 27, getting my shoes on turned into a five-minute saga, with heavy breathing, taking small breaks, and the occasional expletive.

Something had to change.

Eyeing a flyer for a Yoga class just a 20-minute walk from my work, I called the number and spoke to a yoga teacher. I asked her what type of Yoga it was, and she told me it was Bikram Yoga. Pretending to have a clue what she was talking about, I boasted about my background in dance, though I actually hadn't danced since I was 15.

I think she believed me. Phew.

Calvin Klein leggings and a T-shirt were all I had to wear. There was no Lululemon, and sports stores were not stocking Yoga apparel yet. I took a big towel to practice on as there were no Yoga mats. When I walked in, I noticed no one else had them.

I waited in the reception area of the Yoga school, which had a studio that was just off to the side. In the class before mine, students started coming out drenched with sweat and using their hands to talk because breathing was all they could muster. Speaking wasn't an option.

Walking into class, the teacher, Suzanne, was sitting on the floor; she was in her late 40s, perhaps 50s. It was hard to tell as her body was youthful and toned and she has a sense of vibrancy behind her eyes. Suzanne was sitting in Dragon Fly pose, with a cash tin and notebook in front of her.

I reminded Suzanne who I was with the hope my story of athleticism dance would jog her memory of our call. Politely, she smiled, nodded, and told me to stand at the back. The room filled. She started with a breathing exercise and everyone seemed to know what they were doing. Trying my best, I pretended to know what I was doing. Hearing lots of strange sounds emitting from people's mouths, it sounded like a swarm of locusts.

The Yoga class was 90 minutes. It seemed short, hot, hard, and painful. Instantly, I was addicted and hurried home to let my boyfriend know all about my new hobby.

The next day, I was back on the mat with my towel and reused juice container filled with three liters of water. I put my towel down and lay on top in Savasana waiting for class to start.

Practicing four times per week, I plunged deeper in love with Yoga. When I was at parties, I would corner other guests to tell them all about this new hot Yoga I was doing and how amazing I was feeling.

Nothing in my life had made me feel this good; not drugs, alcohol, love, or any life experience. **NOTHING.**

After September 11th, 2001, with the terrorist attacks on the World Trade

Center, I decided to quit my job in corporate, head back home, and do Yoga teacher training. The world was in limbo, and I was worried World War II was going break out.

In September 2002, I embarked on the intensive Bikram Yoga Teacher Training in Los Angeles. It was the most grueling, hellish, amazing journey I've ever embarked on.

After training, I felt bulletproof.

In 2003, I was teaching all around Sydney. When I first arrived in January, Bikram Hot Yoga was booming. New studios were popping up everywhere. Feeling I had finally found my niche, I left Sydney full of excitement and possibilities and returned to Adelaide wanting to build my first Bikram studio.

In Adelaide, the massive changes sunk in while away in L.A. and Sydney for two years. My relationship crumbled as we were both going on a different trajectory. Do I return to L.A. and work on faculty for Teacher Training? Move back to Jersey? Back to corporate? Back to Sydney? Teach for other studios?

I decided to stay in Adelaide and continue on my quest to open a studio. With the resolution of my relationship, I came out worse for wear financially. I had already found a space upstairs from a restaurant that was perfect for a studio. It needed a lot of work, but I had a great builder with a "can do" attitude. Spending a lot on getting my studio through council approval, it was weeks away from having the application formally accepted.

One morning, I received a call from my former coworker, Freyer. She was recently divorced and looking for something new. We discussed where I was with my new venture, and her desire to become a teacher. We even talked about doing the studio together. Shortly after that, we formed a company together and built the first Bikram Yoga studio.

My accountant said....

"It won't work, Yoga in the 40-degree heat, for 90 minutes. It's a huge risk and massive capital outlay."

But I knew firsthand how much Yoga changed my life, and I knew I could help others.

It was going to work, and we opened a studio in May 2004. By the end of the first year, we did renovations. Having numerous students become teachers, we decided to add more classes. A year later, I traveled to Perth and looked for space to open our second studio. It was there that I became pregnant and came back home to Adelaide to have my baby.

It soon became clear we had outgrown our original space. Our landlord had another building, with double the space, just five minutes away. The new studio was 7,000 sqft and could fit over 100 students in class.

We now had two receptionists at the desk for our busy classes. There was a section dedicated to retail. We sold everything needed for Yoga and every single brand of coconut water. Hot Yoga was booming, and coconut water was more popular than water. Who thought that the water from this large fruit could produce such hysteria?

During this time, my business relationship with Freyer had come to an end. For me to continue doing what I loved, I had to sell my shares of the studios and downsize my city studio. As the business divorce was harrowing, I got severe depression and could barely function. Had it not been for my son and the Yoga, I really don't know if I would have gotten through.

Frequently, I found myself practicing Yoga with tears streaming down my face. The fear of the unknown, and all the hard work I had done to open studios with a partner was a disaster.

*Telling my students… "The issues are **within** our tissues…"*

All my emotions would bubble to the surface as I practiced. I was processing and releasing so much energy.

Yet, I still returned to my mat no matter what.

The business divorce was a mess and took two years to finalize. Unspeakable words came out, and I knew that through any fear of the unknown, surviving and thriving were the only options. And I did.

I formed a new company in 2021 called One Degree, and there are now three studios. In addition, multiple disciplines of Yoga and Hot Pilates have been introduced. There is a new and growing teacher training program. To top it all off, we have added a virtual platform with worldwide access to take a class at any time.

Yoga has taken me to amazing places, and I've met incredible people all over the world. I will forever be grateful for stumbling upon that purple Yoga flyer that fateful winter morning.

*By the way, **"Oh, The Places You Will Go"** is my favorite book by Dr. Seuss.*

My 3 Tips for You…

1. Go! Start today! Don't wait for next week, month, or when an injury has healed or to lose weight.

2. Avoid large meals before practice. If you must eat, eat fruit.

3. Nobody is looking at you when you practice. Everyone is caught up with their own emotions; keep this in mind when you feel self-conscious.

Who's Amy?

Amy Kreminski is a proud mother of three, partner to Andrew, and Director of One Degree Fitness Studios. Her main focus is on bringing out the best in people by using the principles of mindfulness and wellness. Amy started practicing Yoga in 2001 and became a certified teacher in 2002. Her passion has led to building and selling seven Hot Yoga studios in Australia.

To learn more about Amy Kreminski and all the authors, please visit www.innerpoint.com

Leo Eisenstein

Essay Twenty-Three

"Realization of Self"

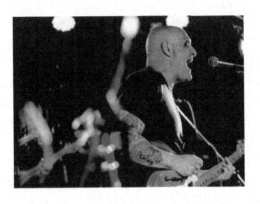

As we get older, the consequences of not taking care of our health can become more obvious, especially when we see family or friends getting sick or dying due to poor health choices. It's a reminder to get yourself in for a much-needed check-up.

For me, visiting a doctor was not going to be comfortable.

Since I was paying for health care anyway, I made the appointment and went to see the doctor. Still, I gained a considerable amount of weight and had fallen into some disrepair.

At the time, I was living a really great life. Essentially, the rock 'n' roll lifestyle. Two years earlier, the band broke up and I had been pretty bummed out. Yet, here I was, finally getting back to feeling like myself— Leo. I was happy with my job and in my relationship, and I was comfortable with my lifestyle. Working in a bar at the time, I was living a pretty plush life. There was a lot of drinking, smoking, and eating out, plus partying till all hours of the night.

Dr. Lang was the doctor to all of the South Street denizens in Philly, where I am from. Having treated so many of my friends, there was an air of familiarity that made our visit very comfortable. The initial check-up went relatively smoothly. She took some blood and weighed me. She gave me the once over and without saying much, sent me on my way.

Three weeks later, I went for a follow-up visit and Dr. Lang wasn't happy in the least. My cholesterol was at 352 and my triglycerides were over 400. The scales were tipping at a whopping 418 pounds. After much finger wagging, she suggested I affect what she referred to as a drastic immediate behavioral change.

UGH... so much for the rock 'n' roll lifestyle.

Her first suggestion seemed too simple. Stop drinking endless glasses of soda. After just three weeks, I went back and had already lost 18 pounds.

Could it be that simple?

She put me on a diet regimen that was a huge change to the way that I had been eating. But I knew that if I was going to help myself, it was time to get real. Believing the hard work would pay off, I was all in.

After losing about 40 pounds, a plateau had been reached and nothing much was changing. Never being much for exercise myself, Dr. Lang suggested that it was indeed the next step in getting my health back. Playing various sports growing up, I detested practice, though liked the games. The gym pretty much sucked, though occasionally, I would ride a bike if I needed to get somewhere. Never would I ride just for the fun of it. It was much better to hang around and smoke, drink, and watch TV.

You know, the fun stuff...lol.

Wait a minute, maybe there was some type of exercise I could do. For some time, my wife had been doing this crazy hot Bikram Yoga. It had made a fantastic and remarkable change in her. First, it made a slender person more fit. Second, it seemed to transfer her overall outlook and make her glow even more.

If Yoga could take a person who's in good shape and make them in better shape, what would it do for someone that is in miserable shape?

After some prodding and convincing, mostly by myself **to** myself, it was time to take my first class. To say the least, it was a nightmare. I left the class at least three times to rinse off in the shower. But since I was absolutely determined, I went back in. There was no way I could let something get the better of me.

No way.

Quickly, I started to notice what it was doing for me. I kept going to more classes. I went to class after class. Then another class...

... and then another class.

I ended up in the tutelage of a very encouraging teacher named Joel Pier, who, at the time, was the studio director at a yoga studio in Philadelphia. He taught everyone how to see Yoga as a discipline, not an exercise. The focus on the outside of my body gave me an awareness of what I was putting in my body. Not just the food, but the thoughts going into my mind. Forming the ability to change my mind, I began to feel different about myself. A daily practice became the norm.

The changes were immediate and remarkable.

Adding a 90-minute hot Yoga routine to my life made such an unbelievable difference. Friends and other people began to notice something had changed.

The good doctor kept testing my liver enzymes to see if they were being affected by the statins that she put me on for high cholesterol. Was the protocol actually doing any good or was damage being done to my liver? At that point, it was still unclear.

We started talking about this crazy Yoga I was doing virtually every day. Diving into all the health benefits of the practice, I asked her if I could drop the statins. She said if I continued the blood tests, why not? The commitment to my health and my practice was continuing to get stronger.

In less than two years, my cholesterol plummeted from 352 to 178, and with true amazement, 228 pounds fell off my body. It was the first time in decades that the scales tipped in at only 190 pounds. None of it was easy, though worth every drop of sweat to get me there.

The motivation to continue now comes from within.

When you decide for yourself, you can maintain a healthy weight and stay in healthy shape through your personal commitment and awareness of your own self. You can decide to be in control of your destiny.

Not just speaking about physical health, but mental health, emotional health, and spiritual health as well. Only if someone can stop long enough to see themselves in the mirror will they start noticing the person standing in front of it.

The realization of the self is the true value of your life.

I'm not saying this is for everyone, but I am saying that it worked for me and I can tell you that the healing benefits of Yoga cannot be denied.

Truly leaving the rock 'n' roll lifestyle behind and deciding to become a teacher opened my eyes to the dedication and rigors of living the Yoga lifestyle. After a vigorous 10 weeks of intensive teacher training in 2005, the path and journey in my life changed.

It's an honor and pleasure that at over 60 years old, I'm actually able to teach about 20 classes a week. As time goes on, there's this strong thirst for knowledge about how Yoga works. Not just the postures themselves, but what's going on inside the mind and the spirit. In the end, this is where the real work is.

Being big, bald, and tattooed was only the start of it.

Yoga can help you through the crisis of the deaths of friends and family members. Raising children can become delightful, even with all the pitfalls life seems to throw at you. Through regular practice, a place of refuge is ready to open inside of you. Growing physically, mentally, and spiritually becomes effortless.

Regardless of what you do, can you be inspired to go within?

I invite you to ask yourself if you're living the life that you truly want. Is there something you want to change? Are you willing to take the step to make it happen?

Hint: When you're ready, it can happen relatively quickly!

My 3 Tips for You...

1. Be the catalyst for your own change.

2. Try to look for the good in everything, not just the things that you like. You will start to notice that there's goodness all around.

3. Never say never.

Who's Leo?

Leo is a big bald tattooed, former bartender/hockey player from Philly. He lived a lot of life before he found himself at a crossroads. It was either make a turn for the worse or make a turn for the better. He chose better! Leo began his Yoga practice in 2002 and today teaches as much as he possibly can.

To learn more about Leo Eisenstein and all the co-authors, visit www.innerpointe.com.

Kay Forrester

Essay Twenty-Four

"Find Your Agape"

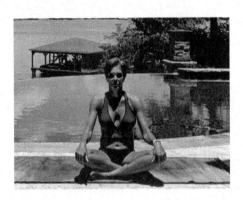

The definition of AGAPE is Sacrificial Love, the highest form of Love that exists!

Agape is given without any expectations of receiving anything in return. When you selflessly and unconditionally help others understand their truest and highest potential (self-realization), this is a form of Agape. When the people you help do the same for someone else, life changes for everyone!

During childhood, I knew there was something special I needed to do in my life. I daydreamed of being a cowgirl or a movie star and traveling. I remember making a salt and flour map of the United States and being curious about Washington State, a place far away from the small rural town in Georgia, where I am from.

My father was a home builder. He was meticulous and rarely subcontracted work. My mother was a teacher's aide and school lunchroom supervisor. She was adventurous and loved to cook and travel. I had humble beginnings but learned something special from each of them!

Eager to discover what life had to offer, I accelerated my studies in school. I wasn't particularly athletic but enjoyed sports. Personally, I found more satisfaction in 4-H, an educational program focusing on leadership, citizenship, public speaking, and life skills. Their motto is:

"To Make the Best Better!"

So, I pledged:

"My Head to clearer thinking, My Heart to greater loyalty, My Hands to larger service, and My Health to better living for my club, my community, my country, and my world!"

In 4-H, my yearly project was raising and selling show cattle. My parents helped with expenses, but I earned enough money to study abroad for a summer. For this, I received credit for early college admission and attended summer school to finish my business degree before I turned 20.

After graduation, I went to work for an electric utility company where my job was to help residential and commercial customers become more energy efficient. Later, I married my high school sweetheart, and we spent the next few years working hard and playing hard on Lake Sinclair before having two beautiful children.

In 1996, my husband was offered an assignment in the Northwest, so we moved to Washington State. To stay active, I took a job with a global communications company until things got too busy with my kids. As they got older, I began to wonder what was next. Going back to corporate America, where I spent 19 years of my life, wasn't high on my list.

There had to be more!

In 2009, a friend asked me to go with her to a Bikram Yoga class. I made every excuse not to go, but when she gave me a 10-day pass for my birthday, there was no choice. I hated my first class. The teacher kept reminding me to close my mouth and breathe! I swore I would never go back, but as I recovered and began to think more clearly, I made up my mind to try again. Every day, I went back to Yoga and by day 10, I knew I had found something special I needed to do in my life.

I felt a Divine Calling!

Becoming a Yoga teacher and taking this amazing practice to my home community in Georgia, where Yoga was virtually unknown, was my new purpose. My dilemma was that at 47, I was living 3,000 miles away from my hometown and had no clue how to answer the call. *Within,* I could hear my mother saying,

"Where there is a will, there is a way!"

I was unable to stop thinking about this new calling and wishing I had arned about Yoga sooner. I didn't realize prior life experiences would e so important. First, I had to figure out how and when to go to Bikram oga Teacher Training. My kids were still in school, so I planned to keep racticing until they went to college.

hat December, we traveled to Georgia for Christmas and decided to ok for a cabin on Lake Sinclair. We hoped to find a summer retreat but nexpectedly found a perfect retirement home. Our situation was tricky ecause my husband needed to transition work and my kids needed to nish school. Two years later, things fell into place.

Vhen my youngest went to college, I headed to teacher training, which as the perfect empty-nester thing for me to do. I was very apprehensive ecause, at 51, I didn't know if I was capable. There was no Yoga studio ear my home, so I had to prepare by practicing on my own. Fortunately, ne summers were hot enough to practice outside, but I had to improvise uring the cooler months. There were also people in my life who thought I ad lost my mind! Nevertheless, I knew *within*, I had to...

nswer the Call!

ikram Yoga teacher training was where Heaven meets Hell! It was one f the toughest but most gratifying experiences I have ever had. All the ainees endured nine weeks of early mornings, insanely late nights, two xtremely hot classes almost every day, endless lectures, posture clinics, ollywood movies, 47 pages of dialogue memorization, a little Indian man illing us every time he taught class, and his staffers telling us to...

Trust the Process!"

t was physically and mentally exhausting and I was convinced I was going fail!

ne of the requirements at teacher training was to present the "Half loon" pose to Bikram in front of 300+ people and receive his feedback. I as petrified because his feedback could be brutal. I nervously stumbled hrough my presentation, thinking he was going to verbally crucify me, ut he looked me dead in the eye and said,

You are going to help a lot of people!"

le saw something deep *within* me that I never knew existed.

fter training, I was in the best shape of my life, but unfortunately, I didn't eel ready to teach. Determined not to give up, I continued to study yoga nd hone my teaching skills for the next six weeks.

My first teaching gig was in a beautiful studio in Birmingham, Alabama. When I arrived for my interview, the studio owner asked me to teach! I was terrified and had nothing to wear, so I purchased a new Yoga outfit in the studio and headed for the podium to teach. I struggled through class and was certain I had let everyone down! After class, with my head hung low, I met with the studio owner. She looked at me with the kindest eyes and said,

"You are exactly where you need to be!"

After two years of traveling and teaching, it was time for me to open a studio in the small college town where I lived. Incidentally, the carpentry skills learned from my dad and the knowledge gained from working with heating and air conditioning contractors while in the energy business were essential for the project!

Opening a Hot Yoga studio was risky in my demographic because I would have to teach people what Yoga is and explain the benefits, before teaching them how to do postures and practice. Rumors were flying and I was the butt of many jokes. Bikram Yoga is still hard to sell in my community, but my people need Yoga, so I help them discover it!

Running a studio requires tremendous time, energy, and money. To stay competitive, I had to get additional training and diversify my offerings. During the Covid-19 pandemic, I had to draw upon my technical and problem-solving skills to stay engaged with my clients. The silver lining was that we were able to produce over 100 videos for my students and have since set up an incredible ZOOM experience to host teachers from around the world.

My Yoga journey started late in life. Yours can too! Yoga has taught me that things happen at the right time, at the right place, and for the right reason. More importantly, I discovered the true meaning of sacrificial love through Yoga. My AGAPE is to serve others by helping as many people as possible discover this life-changing practice.

Remember, God has a Divine plan, and you are exactly where you need to be!

At 60, I practice and teach as much as possible. I want to be an inspiration to my students and for them to see me as their Agape Guide, who falls out of postures and is dedicated to their wellness and mine. I say to my students after every class,

"We rise by lifting others!"

In the words of the late Dr. Martin Luther King Jr.:

"Life's most persistent and urgent question is, 'What are you doing for others?'"

My 3 Tips for You...

1. Where there is a will, there is a way.

2. You are stronger than you think. Answer the call.

3. You are exactly where you need to be. Find your Agape!

Who's Kay?

Kay Forrester is a small-town girl who found Yoga late in life. Her journey took her from practicing to teaching to becoming a studio owner. Her energetic style and passionate delivery leave her students inspired and invigorated! Kay has a natural way of helping students find their edge without feeling overwhelmed or intimidated. Along with good nutrition, she believes that as we age, strength, balance and flexibility are critical for health and well-being. Kay lives by the mantra "If you are strong, healthy and sound of mind, then you can help others. If you can help others help themselves, then you can change the world!"

To learn more about Kay Forrester and all the co-authors, visit www.innerpointe.com.

Spencer James Larson

Essay Twenty-Five

"Just Be"

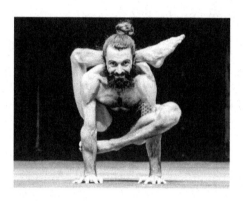

"What do you do?"

While this is a common enough question, it seems that I'm asked this question constantly.

My favorite response is, "Well, I recycle..."

Which always seems to confound or frustrate the one who asked.

The question seems harmless enough of a common conversation starter, but I've always been keenly aware of the judgment with which the question is asked. The question is inherently based on agreed-upon societal constructs: level of education, successes, net worth, a checklist of, "should's," "haves," or your value to society.

That which defines you limits you, and I AM not a job.

You simply cannot SEE me through the lens of this question, and herein lies the Maya; the illusion, the egoic identification of self as separate, placing the value of one human over another in a way that relates time to money; again, constructs. Spiritual aspirants say it is this illusion that they seek to overcome; to which I say, one way to overcome this illusion of separateness IS going *within* through the practice of YOGA.

"JUST BE."

Born in Eugene, Oregon, my childhood was heavily influenced by competitive team sports. As a naturally gifted athlete, there was some strife within me with respect to the pressure and expectations put on me by myself and others—there it is again; the summation of value based on my performance or the outcome of the game, what I did, or how I did. My response to this influence would point me in the direction of my life's path.

Early on in my life, I was shown the light, shown the way, and in my own words, 'SHOWN GOD.' What this means is that I came to know myself and my true nature as peaceful, simple, minimalistic, silent, and still. I'm highly sensitive to energy and vibration, deeply attentive to details in ways that can be interpreted as both precisely mathematical and purely artistic; as present, conscious, and most importantly FREE...

FREE from man-made constructs,

FREE from societal norms,

FREE from having to actually do anything to prove myself and my value,

FREE from even the idea that my value has to be credentialed, earned, argued for, defended, or protected; or that I should have to convince anyone of it based on their measures.

This essence of freedom, inborn, remembered, and ignited, led me to have deeper realizations that my greatest experience of freedom is actually deeply embedded at the core of my being. My priority in life is peace, within and without.

Peace for me is comprised of simplicity, silence, freedom, and nature.

Eventually, skateboarding, snowboarding, solo alpine mountaineering, full moon vision quests, and creating art would become life-changing for me. For more than a decade, I routinely summited the Three Sisters Mountains in Oregon: Hope, Charity, and Faith.

My ascents were strategically planned to reach each peak for perfectly timed sunsets, sunrises, full moons, and eclipses, oftentimes climbing through the gnarliest of storms, traveling mostly in the dark of night on starlit trails. I was literally tapping into extra-sensory powers and developing night vision.

Although I've lost count of how many full moon journeys I've been on, what I discovered is that nature is my true teacher. Her rhythms and cycles align deeply with my own. Her elemental silence makes no demand upon me except that I should be true to and present with myself in my solitude, in my silence, in my freedom and peace.

What do you do to know yourself as free?

While adventuring on the island of Kauai, I picked up the book *Autobiography of a Yogi* by Paramahansa Yogananda, which in a way led me to take my first Yoga class. I felt divinely guided and incredibly blessed to walk out of my job and into my first Bikram Hot Yoga class on August 8, 2008, in Bend Oregon.

I delight in saying, "I learned to bend in Bend." By now, having accumulated multiple serious injuries from the amount of fun and adventure I was partaking in, I found this hot class to be in perfect resonance with my inner knowing and my inner-peace priority.

Not only did this scientific method of health help to heal my body, but it also got me back on the mountain, back on the snowboard, back into the mid-air freedom of expression through connection to nature which had become my life. And for the first time, it put a mirror before me. Literally, the mirror invited me to see what I had already known, what others feel they have to work to find or earn; and that is that I AM and GOD IS.

What can you do to JUST BE?

Yoga competition. Standing on the X. A demonstration of mastery of the central nervous system. A three-minute journey of the self, through the self, to the self.

In the yoga competitions, I will say that my natural style was, "to not try too hard." As you know about me by now, having to try too hard was what I had let go of early on in my quest for peace. Further, I had embraced self-compassion which was the earnest requirement of the injuries I had sustained over time. I would stand on stage, on the X spot, over 13 times in the ensuing 13 years. Feeling blessed, I received the gold medal for the United States of America on August 8, 2021, 13 years to the day of my first yoga class.

Even more auspiciously, I had the honor of representing the USA in the International Yoga Sports Federation World Championship of Yogasana Sports in Bangalore, India in 2022. There, a group of IYSF's recent champions, including myself, were graced with the invitation to demonstrate for the Prime Minister of India for the greatest Spectacular Event of the World Yogasana Championships to date!

How do you connect to the cosmic consciousness?

After adventuring through Israel and Egypt came a couple of years of diligent practice in preparation to one day attend Teacher Training. Before attending the two-month-long teacher training, I made my first of several adventures to the Motherland of Yoga to attend the largest gathering of humanity at once during the 2013 Maha Kumbh Mela, together with my lifelong friend. There, I found myself running naked through the streets with the Naga Babas to the main bathing place upon sunrise. This was a truly sacred and profound experience for me.

For my friend, the experience of the Mela was that of complete overwhelm, chaos, and fear; but for myself, it was one of inner peace—the calm in the eye of the storm. There among over 120 million people in attendance during the course of 55 days, and what did I do? JUST BE.

What can you do to experience calm in the eye of the storm?

After the Mela came the adventure to Bikram Yoga Teacher Training in the spring of 2013 in Los Angeles. I drove my dad's VW van down from Oregon, loaded up with bulk supplies, superfoods, a hot plate, and Vitamix. While the physical challenge was intense, the more difficult challenge for me was committing a 40-page script to memory.

I've been incredibly blessed to have been able to take my teaching skills worldwide, eventually landing on the Big Island of Hawaii for a while, where I like to say, I taught myself how I wanted to teach.

I immersed myself in my teaching, in love, in the waters, in the black, red, green, and white sand beaches. I watched the Earth being formed as liquid hot lava poured into the ocean. I dove off cliffs and waterfalls, foraged for my food, flew helicopters, went skydiving, lived off the grid on the most incredible coffee farm, meditated on Mauna Kea, and sun gazed for countless evening hours in Kona town.

Can you see now how 'What do you do?' just doesn't quite cut it?

Returning to the mainland in 2018, unsure of my next move, I road-tripped on my Ural motorcycle with my two dogs in the sidecar for seven weeks. Along the way, I taught and practiced wherever I could, all up and down the West Coast. I got back on the stage for the USA Yoga and IYSF Competitions and attended multiple seminars to raise the bar on my teaching and understanding of the postures.

As fate would have it, I found myself in the High Desert of Southern California, where in the most ironic and iconic of ways, every aspect of my life—every skill I've picked up along the way, every vision I've held and desire that I've had to create a Sanctuary, a Healing Arts and Spiritual Sciences Yoga and Event Center—has become a material reality.

I create Vibrational Art. I host Yoga Retreats and Sound Baths. I do breath work. I co-lead a Spiritual Study group, and I facilitate Quantum Healing by supporting people in DEEP SEE DIVES through Private Plant Medicine Ceremonies at Yucca Shala.

Yucca Shala is a Healing Arts Sanctuary and Retreat Center for all things Yoga and Spirit. An incredible co-creation and collaboration of epic proportion with my beloved, where we delight in nourishing others on every level of BE-ing. All are WELCOME, please come visit.

My 3 Tips for You...

1. Learn to walk upon the Earth as if your feet are kissing it with each step you take.

2. Spend time in nature; learn how to see and realize that everyone and everything is connected.

3. And yes, finally... "JUST BE."

Who's Spencer?

Spencer James Larson is a Visionary Artist, an Extreme Gravity Sport Enthusiast, Solo Alpine Mountaineer, Snowboarder, Golfer, International Yoga Instructor, Sound Medicine Practitioner, Modern day Mystic and Plant Medicine Guide. Spencer found Yoga to be incredibly beneficial not just for the body, but also the mind. After years of cultivating a regular Yoga practice, he became a teacher in 2013. Spencer is Co-Creator and Proprietor of Yucca Shala, a small Private Event Center for the Healing Arts and Spiritual Sciences located in the high desert of Southern California.

To learn more about Spencer Larson and all the co-authors, visit www.innerpointe.com.

Balwan Singh

Essay Twenty-Six

"Even Warriors Get Knocked Down"

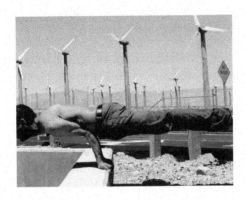

Even though I grew up in a warrior class cast/family in Rishikesh, India, I could not discover any of my strengths or gifts throughout my early life. Struggling throughout my childhood, I was constantly worried about the future. Waking up every morning, I remember I used to think to myself... *how far can I push myself?*

It affected my self-confidence and perspective about the outside world. We are all supposed to discover our special talents, but I could not find a single gift.

Perhaps, I was looking in the wrong place.

Life has its own mysterious ways to knock you down even if you think you are the biggest warrior ever. Yoga and self-discipline provide you with the antidote. When you least expect it, life teaches you the most precious lesson. I got a taste of courage through struggles and experiences later in life. The secret to getting ahead in life is to get started. If something is important to us, our minds will always find ways to achieve it against all odds.

We are all gifted in our own way.

True happiness and contentment come when we use our talent to make money and share it with the world. Every person has to find a way to share their talent with the world. Nobody knows the best way to deliver your unique idea—other than you.

Winning response

We live in a world of infinite possibilities. I grew up in a small village where electricity and freshwater were a luxury and of course, it was not available to us. It wasn't until fourth grade that I first saw a motor car. We had everything except money and materialistic things. Because we were too busy carrying loads of books and pleasing others, we did not realize the importance of yoga or physical exercise.

The challenge is not to manage time, but to manage ourselves. Peace of mind comes when your life is in harmony with true principles and values

Is there a book that has inspired you?

Swami Vivekananda inspired and moved me from the beginning. The most life-changing lines were, "Take up one idea. Make that one idea your life—think of it, dream of it, and live on that idea. Let the brain, muscles, nerves, every part of your body be full of that one idea, and just leave every other idea alone."

This is the way to lead a successful life.

Our brain is wired to compete and judge.

If we keep working on developing a little bit every day, it creates massive results and we become more valuable to ourselves and others. The idea is to break the task into smaller measurable chunks. Just like in a yoga practice, big rewards come from small and seemingly insignificant actions.

Timing is a huge factor.

A large factor that contributes to our success in life can often be the difference between complete failure and monumental success. We have to continue learning how to use our time more productively; to free up time for making things that are important to us.

Things like single-tasking, smaller projects, tracking your progress, setting goals, doing timed work sessions free of interruption, and adding accountability are all proven methods for maximizing our productivity in a short amount of time. Often, when you have less time to get something done, you become more productive.

Law of cause and effect

When one door of happiness closes, another opens. Everything happens or a good reason. At one time many years ago, I thought I had the most meaningful and powerful dream job working at Bikram Yoga Headquarters to teach the trainings. Everything comes to end someday. Out of a surprise, the job simply ended. I felt like I was at square one again.

Even though I thought I was the most influential and powerful person n the Yoga world, inside I felt empty, and that I lacked accomplishment. We are only able to connect the dots when moving forward. Mild success can come to us through skills and hard work, but wild success is usually attributable to being present at the right time and right place.

Necessity is a great teacher.

Each of us is born with unique gifts and valuable talents. When we share our gifts with others, we often feel the happiest and most content. This is the purpose of life, *to simply be happy*. Many answers quickly reveal themselves when we take the first step.

Everything we do along the journey contributes to our goals and success. Our thoughts and beliefs dictate our reality. After many failed attempts, I was able to find a new career that could pay my bills and generate an income to support my family. But it came with a cost, and that was less time to regularly teach yoga classes and practice as much as I like.

Everything in life is an invention.

In 2014, I went to Pune, India to meet Yogi and author B.K.S. Iyengar. In spite of being born in India, I felt like an alien in his presence. It was as if I was in a different world.

When you pay for something in India, the product or services are not guaranteed. There are no complaint boxes or Yelp reviews; you are completely at the mercy of God. Through this struggle in my home country, the idea of YogaTalk Global was born; a community where all our voices matter.

It was important to me to build an organization where people can find trustworthy service and feel connected with the worldwide Yoga community. Wealth has then become the result of reliable service and consistent efforts.

Discovering the West

Coming from India, when I moved to the West, I realized the big difference in both cultures and how people respond to various events. All of us have many maps in our minds; maps of the way things are, or realities, and maps of the way things should be, or values.

Through these mental maps, we interpret everything we experience. It's easy to simply assume that the way we see things is the way they really are or the way we think they should be. When in reality, each of us looks through the screen of our own life and perceptions. As such, what we see is often not real.

Each of the essays in this book holds ideas you can use. The answer is not to look outside of ourselves to determine who we are, but as all the great masters say, *look within*. This is where you'll find everything you need.

My Three Tips for You...

1. Take time to appreciate your own strengths. You become more valuable by working on your strengths.

2. Win through your actions and behavior, not through your arguments. Learn to become a better listener. Practice reading other people's emotions. The more you can understand how people express emotions, the more you will understand other people.

3. The more you develop your personal practice, the more you are connected to source energy and deepen your intuition. Focus on what makes you feel good. The better your body feels, the happier and more productive you are.

Who's Balwan?

Balwan Singh is the founder of the YogaTalk Global Community and YogaTalk Events. He has been involved in teaching trainings internationally for the past 14 years. His engineering background offers a structured and scientific approach to yoga postures and philosophy. Presently he is working full time as a Data Architect for AT&T and teaching yoga classes part-time as a guest teacher.

To learn more about Balwan Singh and all the co-authors, visit www.innerpointe.com.

"No one outside ourselves can rule us inwardly.

When we know this,
we become free."

~ Buddha

Conclusion

The subject of this book is not about mindfulness, breathing, meditation, walking, Yoga, or any other tools for life. It is not about any of the 20 revealing essays about other people's experiences. As mentioned in the Introduction, **the purpose of this book is to help you realize that you have all the answers you need, _within you_.** The subject of this book is about the object—<u>YOU.</u>

Yes, by having read through each of the essays, you now have a pretty good idea of how others have done it, and how going _within_ can help _you_ create your most incredible life ever. It doesn't matter what your life looks like now—by making a decision, you have the power to change it whenever you want.

A life well-lived can be measured in many ways, but the most significant is the impact one has had on others during their time on this earth. Achievements and successes can be important, but _what truly matters is the difference one has made in the lives of those around them._

Over the course of a lifetime, each of us has the opportunity to touch countless lives and leave behind a lasting legacy that will be remembered for generations. By living a life that is guided by kindness, compassion, and service to others, all of us can create an ongoing ripple effect that will extend far beyond our own time on this earth.

Life is not without its challenges and setbacks. But it is often through adversity and hardship that one can grow and learn, developing resilience and tenacity that allows us to continue pushing forward despite so-called obstacles. By facing our challenges with courage and grace, we can inspire others to do the same and leave behind a legacy of strength, perseverance, and _love_.

As the years pass and one reflects _within_, the memories that stand out the most are those that were shared with loved ones and the moments of joy and connection that make life truly worth living. Whether it is a family vacation, a special occasion, or simply spending time together, it is these moments that one treasure most and remembers fondly.

In a nutshell, a meaningful life is one that is guided by love, compassion, and service to others. During our short time on earth, each of us can impact countless lives and leave behind a legacy that will be remembered for generations. By going _within_ and embracing challenges with grace and cherishing moments of joy and connection, Yoga and other simple tools can create a life that is rich in meaning and purpose, and truly worth living.

Perhaps the biggest life I've had in life is this...

Whatever it is, don't worry about it, just live your life.

Michael Harris

To learn more about our authors, programs and retreats, visit us at www.innerpointe.com

References & Citations

Dr. Avi Sharma
Essay Two
References

1. 1). Physical Activity and Incident Depression: A Meta-Analysis of Prospective Cohort Studies; Felipe B Schuch et al; The American Journal of Psychiatry, 2018

2. 2). Rapid stimulation of human dentate gyrus function with acute mild exercise; Kazuya Suwabe et al; PNAS Journal 2018

3. 3). The Joy of Movement. How exercise helps us find Happiness, Hope, Connection, and Courage. Book by Kelly McGonigal

4. 4). Principles and Practice of Yoga in Health Care. Book by Sat Bir Khalsa, Lorenzo Cohen, Timothy McCall, Shirley Telles

5. 5). Breath: The New Science of a Lost Art. Book by James Nestor

Rowena Jayne, ND
Essay Five
References

1. Campbell KA. The neurobiology of childhood trauma, from early physical pain onwards: as relevant as ever in today's fractured world. Eur J Psychotraumatol. 2022 Oct 18;13(2):2131969. doi: 10.1080/20008066.2022.2131969. PMID: 36276555; PMCID: PMC9586666

2. Schneiderman N, Ironson G, Siegel SD. Stress and health: psychological, behavioral, and biological determinants. Annu Rev Clin Psychol. 2005;1:607-28. doi: 10.1146/annurev.clinpsy.1.102803.144141. PMID: 17716101; PMCID: PMC2568977.

3. Harsanyi S, Kupcova I, Danisovic L, Klein M. Selected Biomarkers of Depression: What Are the Effects of Cytokines and Inflammation? Int J Mol Sci. 2022 Dec 29;24(1):578. doi: 10.3390/ijms24010578. PMID: 36614020; PMCID: PMC9820159.

4. Macy RJ, Jones E, Graham LM, Roach L. Yoga for Trauma and Related Mental Health Problems: A Meta-Review With Clinical and Service Recommendations. Trauma Violence Abuse. 2018 Jan;19(1):35-57. doi: 10.1177/1524838015620834. Epub 2015 Dec 9. PMID: 26656487. INTERNET:

Inner*pointe*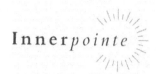

"We all have the power to transform our lives and find true happiness *within*. Innerpointe offers practical transformative approach's to uncovering your inner wisdom and unlocking your full potential. Whether you're struggling with relationships, health, career, or simply feeling unfulfilled, discover ancient wisdom for today's world, that can help guide you towards a deeper understanding of yourself and the world around you.

Through powerful exercises, thought-provoking questions, and inspiring stories from real people, Innerpointe provides personal step-by-step roadmaps and frameworks for personal growth and self-discovery. By committing to this journey, you will gain the tools and insights needed to overcome obstacles, tap into your intuition, and create the life you truly desire.

Don't wait any longer to live your best life. Join the Innerpointe movement today and start your journey towards true happiness and fulfillment.

Visit www.innerpointe.com now and discover the power within you.

Made in USA - North Chelmsford, MA
1372188_9781666402490
06.07.2023 1738